Critical

Critical

Why the *NHS* is being betrayed and how we can fight for it

Dr Julia Grace Patterson

MUDLARK

Mudlark
HarperCollins*Publishers*
1 London Bridge Street
London SE1 9GF

www.harpercollins.co.uk

HarperCollins*Publishers*
Macken House, 39/40 Mayor Street Upper
Dublin 1, D01 C9W8, Ireland

First published by Mudlark 2023

1 3 5 7 9 10 8 6 4 2

© Dr Julia Grace Patterson 2023

Dr Julia Grace Patterson asserts the moral right to
be identified as the author of this work

A catalogue record of this book is
available from the British Library

ISBN 978-0-00-860349-6

Printed and bound in the UK using 100%
renewable electricity at CPI Group (UK) Ltd

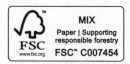

For my sun, my moon and all the stars, MDP

'Medicine is a social science, and politics is nothing else but medicine on a large scale.'
Rudolf Virchow

CONTENTS

AUTHOR'S NOTE

I am a medical doctor by background, and I worked in the NHS for the best part of a decade. But I'm not working clinically any more. Instead, I've devoted myself to advocating for NHS patients and staff, and fighting for the future of the NHS.

The NHS is in the worst crisis of its 75-year history, and it is not a crisis that has happened by accident. This crisis has been caused by the decisions of politicians. Their decisions, to fragment the service, to overload the staff, to allow the infiltration of private companies into our public healthcare system and to cut the funding, have led to the collapse of our public healthcare system. There are millions of patients now on NHS waiting lists, the longest waiting lists ever. Many people are unable to access the healthcare that they need, which they pay for through their taxes.

The NHS comprises four separate healthcare systems across the UK. For the purposes of this book, I will be focusing on the NHS in England, because the situation is significantly worse there than in the other three nations.

CRITICAL

This is not a history book about the NHS. It's also not a policy book, explaining the intricacies of every NHS reform. It's a book explaining where we are, how it has happened and what needs to happen next.

I have been compelled to write this book as a campaigner. I speak to hundreds of thousands of NHS patients and staff online. I'd like to tell you what I've learned, and what I think we need to do now together, if we would like the NHS to survive for another 75 years. If you have picked this book up, the chances are that you are already worried about what is happening. Welcome on board. We have no time to lose.

Ju

INTRODUCTION

The NHS is an institution. But it's also a political football, kicked back and forth between politicians for the past 75 years. It's a burden to some, and a potent vote-winner for others. It's a construct, framed in the media. It's a set of ideas and a logo. It's a workplace for many and the birthplace of almost all of us. It's become a valued part of our society, it is extraordinarily special, and it's being destroyed. Quietly, intentionally, steadily and cleverly, the NHS is being dismantled by politicians who do not want the NHS to exist in its original form, as a publicly funded, publicly run service aiming to provide equal care for all. Instead, it is being transformed into a cash cow, to create a steady stream of profit for private corporations, funded by the taxpayer.

This focus, this overarching political mission, has been a relentless project for the past 40 years. The public hasn't been consulted on the dismantlement of the NHS, didn't vote for this, and many are unaware of what's going on. It began slowly, but the incremental changes that weakened the service's integrity have now been coupled with funding cuts that have been so severe that the service is now collapsing. The politicians and others who have been advancing this agenda have engaged in a decades-long campaign of deflection, to avoid the scrutiny of the public gaze. Some of their names will be familiar to you and others won't; operating in the background to further corporate interests before moving on, perhaps to the House of Lords, perhaps elevated to a position elsewhere. Rewarded for their commitment to the cause: the privatisation of the NHS.

Four decades on from the inception of these changes, their intentions are not in doubt. We can see before our very eyes the impact of their decisions, decisions they have made based on self-interest and political gain, which have pulled our public healthcare project away from its original principles. Through their decisions, their compromises, their dereliction of duty towards the public, they have disregarded these aims. And this is why the NHS is collapsing all around us. This is why the waiting lists are the longest they have ever been in history. This is why when people are calling for ambulances at their most vulnerable moments, often they are not arriving on time. Sometimes they are not arriving at all, and many patients are needlessly dying, unable to access the care they need. It is horrifying to recognise that this situation is not an accidental happenstance but the realisation of the political ambitions of many people, over many years.

The politicians have not done this alone of course, and this is part of the reason why many people do not understand what has happened. Politicians have been supported and encouraged by political donors, by acquaintances, by the carefully orchestrated, rage-inducing headlines of media outlets that call attention to the failings in the NHS, but not the causes. Blaming the nurses, or the doctors, or the patients. Weaving narratives of almost-truths upon never-truths and preying on people's vulnerabilities, their fear and their anger to do so, until many people believe a tapestry of incendiary soundbites about the service. A tapestry of nonsense. This tapestry provides an excellent shroud for them to operate behind, doing the real work. Writing the legislation to push through reforms, and meanwhile pulling budgets down to render the service dysfunctional, then barely functional, and then not functional at all. Watching this towering institution that once was robust sway, and then start to topple.

And as it begins to topple, they have swept in at various junctures with the changes made possible through their quiet changes to the legislature. The changes that they claim will improve things. They wring their hands on national TV, professing that they love the NHS, but (careful glance to the camera, world-weary stance, rueful smile), things must change because they simply are not working. They have, in this way, implemented solutions to 'save the NHS' over the past 40 years. They have built an internal marketplace, they have entered into partnerships with the private sector and outsourced services, bought capacity in the private sector at busy times and have even started selling off NHS assets to the private sector, including allowing the sale of large numbers of GP practices to a US healthcare insurance company.

These things have not strengthened the service. They have not marked progress for the NHS project, if progress means more equitable care and a more robust public health service. These changes have pulled the service down an entirely different path; the path of privatisation. And they have done so to the detriment of patients and staff; to everyone who relies upon and is a part of the service.

I didn't know about any of this in 2010, when I qualified from medical school. I was too consumed with thoughts about whether I'd do a good enough job for my patients to have the energy to critique politicians' messaging, or to pay attention to the public discourse surrounding the NHS. I didn't consider myself to be 'political' either. Frankly, I wasn't paying enough attention to what was going on. A few short weeks before I started my first job as a junior doctor, George Osborne 'stepped up to the dispatch box as chancellor of the new coalition government and announced the longest and deepest period of cuts to public service spending since the second world war'.[1]

We were told at the time that there was wastage, and bureaucracy, and that things would be trimmed back to make the NHS more efficient. One campaign poster from 2010 showed David Cameron boldly saying, 'I'll cut the deficit, not the NHS.'[2] I didn't have any context with which to understand the cuts in 2010, because I had only just started working within the service. I didn't identify what was being lost at first. But as the cuts progressed over the next few years, their impact became more and more apparent. It didn't feel like the cuts increased the efficiency within the system; quite the opposite. As the cuts stacked up, the service worsened incrementally. The beds were cut, and we felt those cuts as they came. When you cut the number of hospital beds available, at busy times there is less capacity to admit sick patients, and so the bar at which healthcare staff can admit a patient to hospital rises higher and higher. The situation ends up with healthcare professionals denying in-patient care to a growing number of people who would benefit from it. And for the people who are granted an admission, their time in hospital is kept as short as possible in order to discharge one patient and admit the next into the bed as quickly as possible.

Even in the early years of austerity, there were times when we would have preferred to keep a patient for an extra day or two, to keep an eye on their progress and ensure they were ready to manage when they left hospital. But the pressures stacked up, and as this happened, the urgency with which we were asked to discharge patients and make way for new ones also stacked up. During busy times of the year such as the winter period, when there is a greater burden of respiratory illnesses in the population, the NHS was beginning to creak at the seams. The term 'winter crisis' started to be used regularly around 2013, and as time went on, we came to expect periods of intense pressure during the winter months because of a lack of hospital beds. In total, between 2008/09 and 2020, 32,000 overnight hospital beds were cut in the NHS in England.[3]

In addition to the bed cuts, staff roles were cut too. The funding for some roles was removed, and often when members of staff left the service they weren't replaced. This caused the remaining staff to juggle larger and larger caseloads of patients over time. Our job roles became less specialised and nuanced too. For example, if you stop employing a phlebotomist on a hospital ward, the task of taking blood from ward patients falls to a junior doctor. And the task wasn't limited to simply taking the blood. Any clinical task involves a degree of administration too. During one of my ward jobs as a junior doctor I was told that I would increase efficiency if I wrote out all of the blood forms by hand during the morning ward rounds. But if your head is bent over a pile of forms copying down details, you're not paying attention to your patients as the team walks around the ward. You're not properly hearing what they say and observing their body language, and you're not properly listening to the reaction of senior doctors and absorbing what you must do to help your patients for the rest of that day. When the senior doctors left the wards, to run busy clinics, carry out operations, or assess new patients in A&E, I'd be left, holding a pile of blood request forms and often scratching my head about what my patients needed.

Administrator roles were lost in many areas, and many clinicians had to start writing their own clinic letters to patients or manage appointment diaries because we no longer had the support of an admin team. And this created a lot of tension; if healthcare staff spoke up and complained about these things, we were often met with accusations that we were being precious, or arrogant. But a lot of these changes simply made no sense; administrative tasks are essential and take up a lot of time. If frontline clinicians are sitting in an office typing, they're not with patients providing good healthcare. In a lot of ways, the 'efficiencies' made by the government were actually causing enormous inefficiencies within the system.

If you start to cut away the time a clinician has with their patient, you don't cut away their ability to reach an effective diagnosis or deliver treatment immediately. The time that is cut away first is the minutes when a doctor has a chance to listen to a patient's concerns, and perhaps to explain things again if there are aspects the patient hasn't understood. You cut away the minutes that enable you to walk slowly, with the patient, at their pace, into your clinic room, instead of hurrying and bustling in, giving an air of impatience. These things matter; they allow care to feel holistic and they allow patients more autonomy within their healthcare by offering them the space to properly understand things. We felt those minutes being pared back slowly over time. It felt like the government was gradually excising the care within the system.

Junior doctors move between medical departments regularly in order to gain experience in different areas. And as I moved through different departments, working in paediatrics and surgery, A&E and GP, psychiatry and General Medicine, among others, I saw that the pressure in the service was growing everywhere I went. The problems weren't being caused by one or two failing departments struggling to cope with new processes. The inefficiency caused by the 'efficiency savings' was happening across the board. NHS staff absorbed more and more pressure as time went on. We squeezed in extra patients wherever we could, doing things more hastily, and stayed later and later in the evenings to catch up on paperwork. We watched the sky darken outside hospital windows, knowing we wouldn't get home to our families on time again that evening. Just like yesterday. Just like the day before.

As the austerity years progressed, we tried our best to stretch ourselves thinner and thinner to keep the service going and our patients safe. But over time, the cuts started to create an atmosphere of uncertainty and instability within the system itself. There was the sense that these cuts just kept coming, and we were constantly wondering what would be taken away next. I knew many doctors who began to feel rudderless within a profession that had been their vocation. No one enters medicine thinking it will be an easy path, no medical student is under the illusion that it'll be free of stress and challenges. But there had been a sense when I entered medical school in 2004 that the profession would offer constancy to those dedicated enough to stay the course and work hard. This constancy became eroded amid the cuts; our roles felt more precarious and less patient-focused. It began to feel that we were denying care to those who needed it, and never providing quite enough. Many doctors I knew lost their sense of belonging within the profession and started to move abroad during the austerity years, where they were better supported by their employers. Others chose to leave medicine altogether and pursue other careers. The medical profession hadn't turned out how they thought it would be; they never felt like they were doing enough, and the strain of feeling that way day after day simply became too much.

We spoke about the situation a lot, both with colleagues and with our friends from medical school. Along with the cuts, there were real-terms freezes to our pay. It was hard to acknowledge that we were working harder and harder while absorbing real-terms pay cuts. We worried a lot about what would come next for the service, for our patients and for ourselves. Despite these worries, however, I didn't see the early austerity cuts as part of a wider agenda to dismantle the NHS. I hadn't studied the NHS reforms that had been carried out since the 1980s, and we hadn't been taught about them at medical school. I didn't know much about the infiltration of private providers into the service. I only saw what was in front of me; my patients, my diminishing team, and my inability to provide the sort of care I'd dreamt of when I had embarked upon my medical career. I simply didn't recognise the failures within the service as predictable and preconceived. I naively thought that at some point politicians would become shocked to find that their efficiency savings hadn't worked, and would reverse their decisions.

I lost this naivety during the junior doctor contract dispute, which happened between the BMA (our largest trade union) and the government, and began in autumn 2015. Jeremy Hunt wanted a new contract to be implemented, which would scrap overtime rates for junior doctors in England between the hours 7am and 10pm for every day other than Sunday, while increasing the basic pay within our contracts. Hunt had claimed that the cost impact would be neutral, but the BMA were concerned that the proposed contract would involve an increase in working hours, and a relative cut in pay. The dispute centred on negotiations around pay and conditions, and went on until the summer of 2016, when some concessions were made, but many junior doctors were still very unhappy with the contract.

As a junior doctor, you work incredibly hard. After you leave medical school, you move between a huge number of jobs to gain skills and expertise. This involves moving between locations, moving house regularly, and making and abandoning working relationships again and again, because each training placement lasts between three and twelve months. You're usually on an 'on-call rota' that determines the antisocial hours you'll be working during each job; a rolling rota of 'normal days', nights, weekends and evening shifts (which vary depending on the speciality you're working within). But regardless of the speciality, the work is intense. The hours are long, you're constantly learning, the work is very daunting at times, and in your spare time if you'd like to specialise in a particular area, you have to study for exams. The professional exams across all medical specialities are multiple, gruelling and expensive (and you pay for them yourself; it costs hundreds of pounds for every attempt). The sheer number of antisocial hours that you're working can be isolating too; you miss lots of social events such as birthdays and weddings. When I applied for annual leave for my own wedding, I was told that I 'might be able to get the day off'. One year, I worked every single public holiday. That's the job, and NHS doctors accept it. But it's very hard, and it takes a toll.

Conservative manifesto promises during the 2015 General Election had pledged to provide a '7-day NHS'. The King's Fund later explained that the manifesto promise stemmed from some studies that had suggested that mortality rates were higher among patients admitted to hospital over the weekend rather than during the week.[4] It transpired that the evidence behind this was shaky, and as the *Guardian* reported as our contract dispute came to a close, 'Hunt's persistent reference to a "weekend effect" in hospital care, which he has claimed results in 6,000 people dying every year because they were admitted to hospital at the weekend, has been contentious. It has been challenged by academics, health organisations and MPs.'[5]

Still, amid a heated dispute surrounding our contracts, in which we were attempting to negotiate fair pay and working hours following a long period of pay freezes, links between this 'weekend effect' and junior doctors took hold. There were insinuations that junior doctors were lazy and greedy, and didn't want to go the extra mile to keep patients safe over the weekends, as championed by the government. But these insinuations were ludicrous; we were already working incredibly hard. We were fortunate to have the number of hours we worked stipulated by the European Working Time Directive, which set a maximum number of hours that NHS junior doctors can work within their jobs. However, in practice, the hours allocation was done in terms of averages over a period of many weeks. This meant that there were times when our working hours were incredibly intense. One of my junior psychiatry jobs, for example, involved working seven nights on the trot, thirteen hours in a row, covering a large area and several hospitals and other healthcare facilities. We would drive across the city all night, seeing new patients and assessing emergencies. It was frantic; often I'd get in the car to drive in one direction to see a patient, only to have to turn around mid-journey when a nurse called with a more pressing emergency at the hospital in the other direction. As a foundation doctor, several of my jobs involved working 12-day stretches – you'd work all week, you'd be on call for long shifts over the weekend, then do another full week before a break. When I completed my training rotation in A&E for six months, I worked three weekends out of every five. All of this was absolutely standard. We accepted it as part of our necessary training, but it was very, very hard.

Things are much worse now for the staff working in the NHS. But even back in 2015, as well as the shifts we were allocated, we worked many unpaid hours. If the team was busy or your ward patients needed attention, you didn't walk out of the hospital when your shift time ended. That isn't the culture within medicine, or healthcare in general. NHS staff have always gone above and beyond; the service is held together by goodwill. And even when we weren't at work, it was difficult to switch off. There were many times when I lay awake worrying about my patients, or telephoned the ward to check on something in the middle of the night. You feel responsible for your patients, and that responsibility doesn't end when you walk out of the hospital at the end of the day. And so the insinuations that we weren't working hard enough, or that we didn't care adequately for our patients, really touched a nerve among junior doctors.

The barbed comments from Jeremy Hunt around the 'weekend effect' were accompanied by other attacks within the media. The *Sun* newspaper, for example, coined the term 'moet medics', and they and other publications launched what felt like a series of targeted attacks, focusing on leaders within the profession and our trade union representatives, presenting their 'luxurious lifestyles' and fancy holidays. The *Sun* newspaper was forced to later take down photos of one doctor with an elephant, and on holiday with her husband, after she told the newspaper that 'one trip involved volunteering at a hospital and the other was to visit family'.[6]

The media attacks ramped up as strike action was planned and enacted by junior doctors, and they went on for months. And one of the reasons why these media attacks felt so unbearable was that we were faced with public opinion all day long in our workplaces. Patients would make comments about what they'd read in the newspapers, and would sometimes parrot tabloid headlines as they asked us about the dispute, particularly when they felt frustrated by the NHS and the problems they were encountering within the system. After we'd already endured five years of austerity cuts – of watching our colleagues lose jobs, and the services getting steadily worse for our patients – and had to absorb all of this while working harder and harder to keep the service together, the junior doctor contract dispute formed a lightning rod for the profession.

This situation led to pushback from junior doctors, which I don't think anyone would have anticipated. Doctors aren't primarily motivated by money, and are poorly unionised. We're traditionally pretty weak, as a profession, at advocating for our pay and working conditions (consultant salaries, for example, have dropped in real terms by 34.9 per cent since 2008/09). It's difficult to know whether junior doctors would have unified and gone on to take strike action had we not been vilified and misrepresented in the press for months on end.

Many grassroots projects sprang up at that time to help to explain the realities of the situation to the public. Myself and a close university friend, Dr Georgina Wood, decided to start a choir of doctors and other healthcare workers to create a song about the contract dispute and the threats facing the future of the NHS. We called the choir the National Health Singers, and we brought doctors together from all over the country to record a track called 'Yours',[7] focusing not just on the junior doctor contract, but also on the fact that the NHS belongs to the public and that staff and patients needed to come together to fight for it.

Things moved along, and it was soon announced that the government's own Equality Impact Assessment acknowledged that the government's new junior doctor contract would 'impact disproportionately on women'.[8] And yet, after almost a year of junior doctors coming together, striking, speaking up, and attempting to oppose the government's messaging, in autumn 2016 the government imposed a contract upon junior doctors[9] in England that many of us were unhappy about. It was a heavy blow for us all, and we were left reeling.

The deep politicisation of junior doctors, of our patients and their safety within the service during the contract dispute, shocked me and many other doctors, and it also appalled me that the government was willing to malign junior doctors' reputation so flagrantly in the pursuit of their goal. The government behaved ruthlessly, misrepresented facts to the public, and imposed a contract that negatively impacted on some workers more than others. I found myself wondering, if they were willing to behave in this manner towards one group of NHS staff, what were their intentions towards other staff groups? What was the new agenda with their austerity cuts? And what was their plan for the future of the NHS in general?

I think perhaps if life had carried on as normal, if I'd moved on to the next job as a junior doctor and not had time to pause, then I'd wouldn't have given this situation much more of my time. I probably would have shrugged it off and become consumed again by appointments and long shifts and the usual rhythms of working within the NHS. But this isn't what happened; I had my first baby in the middle of the contract dispute. Those first few months with a new baby are a strange, heady time, where minutes feel like days and days pass in the blink of an eye. Having spent years studying, working long hours and focusing on career goals, suddenly I had great expanses of time to fill. And I filled them with thinking and information-gathering. I wanted to know who was making the decisions that affected the NHS, why and where and how. I wanted to understand how all of the pieces fitted together.

I listened to hours and hours of podcast discussions about the think-tanks, trade unions, political parties, quangos and campaign organisations that influence the NHS, and UK politics in general. I read policy documents and NHS reform Bills while my baby slept, picking up the patterns of language used by different organisations, the buzz words. What they would say, and what they avoided saying. I wanted to get to know the arena of healthcare in all its intricacies, with all of its players. When the same names cropped up again and again within the public discourse around the NHS, I researched those individuals, read their profiles, their backgrounds, found out who had appointed them, how they'd got into their positions of power. I looked into the structure and background of the organisations they worked for, and considered the agenda they were advancing through their work. I started to map out how things had been changed within the NHS over the decades, and how they continued to be changed.

I wanted to understand if other things had also been politicised and misrepresented for political gain, what other situations had seen staff members or patients scapegoated in the pursuit of a goal. And I finally saw the NHS 'austerity' cuts and the junior doctor contract dispute within a broader context; the long-running campaign to introduce privatisation into the NHS. I brought my baby along to meetings, rallies and events, and got involved in projects with brilliant people who had been campaigning for the NHS for many years. I had my second baby 17 months after my first. Because there was so much change happening in my personal life, and because I had two periods of maternity leave close together, I felt slightly detached from my job as a doctor for a little while. But this period of my life had a different impact on me as well. I was limited to the streets around where I lived, because I had a baby and a toddler and no car, and I struggled to get onto public transport with my double pram. The pace of my world slowed down. I noticed things. I became more reliant on the NHS myself, as a pregnant woman, as a new mother, and for my babies' checks and vaccinations. I began to appreciate the service on a different level, and I felt the cuts as a patient too. I was readmitted to hospital with sepsis, a week after giving birth to my first baby. It was the same hospital in which I had trained as a doctor myself, and where my husband was a consultant. I saw a completely different side to the NHS sitting in that hospital bed, seeing the staff work, and feeling the vulnerabilities that a lot of hospital in-patients feel when they're unwell. It gave me a greater appreciation of the worth of our public health service and what, specifically, we were losing through these service cuts.

I became more engaged in reading all sorts of media sources, and I started to pay close attention to the organisations that already existed, and what they were doing to hold the government to account regarding its actions towards the NHS. I began to become extremely frustrated that many of the established medical organisations, the trade unions, the Royal Colleges, weren't speaking up effectively about what the government was doing. They had the platform and influence to push back, and yet they weren't doing so in a meaningful manner. But in time, I came to understand why the traditional medical organisations had been so muted for the preceding four decades. They were, and are, limited in terms of their organisational structure, their processes and their own internal politics. Some of these organisations have charitable status, and so they have limits on how critical they can be of the government.

I began to appreciate, also, that there is a considerable reticence among medical leaders to speak up on an individual level. When they have attempted to speak up against government policy previously, some have been side-lined within important national conversations. National policy areas, particularly those grounded in science and health, really benefit from the expertise of medical voices. This therefore places the medical Royal Colleges and others in a difficult position; if they speak up critically about political decision-making in one area, they may face being excluded in another.

But this is a sympathetic assessment of the situation. Over the years, many leaders in UK healthcare have also stayed silent when they could, and should, have spoken up about poor policy decisions. Some have been rewarded with personal career advancement, and others have found ways to profit from the changes politicians have pushed through. And I imagine that even among those who haven't experienced personal gain in these ways, some have stayed silent because of the intense pressure to uphold the status quo and very real risk of being ostracised should they stick their head above the parapet.

I initially felt deeply disappointed when I realised all of this. But over time I thought about the situation differently. I spoke about the situation with other doctors – friends, colleagues at work, doctors online – and I learned that lots of people were feeling dissatisfied and worried about what was happening in the NHS. We came to the horrible realisation that the situation was going to get worse. You can't keep squeezing and cutting things and underpaying people forever. The NHS is ultimately a huge group of people running a system, and we realised that if nothing changed for the better, eventually that system would crumble. We could see what was going to happen, and we wanted to push back.

Lengthy discussions followed as to how best to respond. Grassroots campaigns took up lots of energy among those already working full-time in the NHS, making it difficult to keep up the momentum necessary to see change occur before exhaustion set in. We had learned through other projects, however, that when doctors spoke up as one for their patients, they were given a voice in the media; perhaps, then, we could influence change if we formed a collective. We were very mindful, though, of the need to preserve the anonymity of any doctor speaking up; it is hard for NHS staff to whistle-blow about problems.

We needed a sustainable solution: an organisation that could react to inaccurate messaging in the press and take up campaign causes, speak up for both patients and staff, lobby politicians for change, and support the staff who were working in difficult conditions. And eventually, after much research and gaining advice from anyone we knew who was even vaguely related to the world of non-profit organisations and civil society, a group of us decided to give it a shot and build a new organisation from scratch. I was able to focus on this myself for a little while because of an opportunity that presented itself unexpectedly.

I was coming to the end of the first half of my psychiatry specialist training, a natural break in the training schedule. My husband and I were struggling to afford childcare for our one- and two-year-old children, because we were living in central London and the costs were extremely high and our working hours very long. Paying for childcare that begins at 7.30am, for example, is extremely expensive. We had been wondering whether we should leave London. But we were reluctant to do so; it was our home and my husband had a job he loved in a central London teaching hospital. But when my father-in-law suddenly told us he planned to sell his little cottage in rural Ireland, it hit us both that if we moved there temporarily, our cost of living would decrease significantly and I would be able to focus on this new project while my husband worked away for a while. And so we bought the cottage, I paused working clinically, and we started to spend a lot of time in Ireland. The childcare costs were just a quarter of what they'd been in London. It was lonely, because my husband was away a lot. But it gave me space to think and plan, liaising with the other doctors who were forming the team.

Before it became the norm due to the COVID-19 pandemic, our team of doctors from various grades and specialities found ways to interact with one another remotely. I flew back to London whenever I could, to meet people and set about building and launching our new non-profit organisation. My friend Georgina became the other director, and early in 2019, together with the team, launched EveryDoctor. The name echoes the term 'everyman', our intention being to hold the government to account by drawing attention to the common experiences of frontline doctors, particularly the systemic problems being caused by the governmental cuts, which were causing unsafe and unfair situations for patients and staff.

Systemic problems tend to occur in multiple places by their very nature; when pressures upon the service increase and one NHS workplace encounters problems (for example, due to a lack of paediatric beds or its A&E department experiencing high demand), similar services will likely be under intense pressure somewhere else too. We were fed up of seeing staff or services scapegoated because of problems that were happening due to the cutbacks from the government and the associated pressures. We therefore realised that if we highlighted situations occurring in patterns, systemic problems cropping up in multiple NHS workplaces at the same time, we could hold the government to account for what was happening. We could demonstrate to the public that when problems occurred it wasn't because of one poor hospital or a few poor local leaders; it was because the system was becoming unworkable and required invest-ment and policy changes.

And so we set up an encrypted email address and got started, collating testimony from doctors all over the UK about what was happening, verifying sources, and feed-ing this information to journalists who we had started to link up with. We started slowly, attracting members to the organisation gradually as doctors became aware of what we were doing and wanted to get involved. We had a lot to learn, but we were lucky enough to link up with several investigative journalists who taught us how to keep material safe and secure, and how to safely anonymise our sources. We learned how the media func-tioned, and how to secure publicity and to speak up for patients and staff.

When we started working on the idea, I had imagined that my break from the NHS would be temporary, and I hoped to return to my work as a psychiatry doctor. However, even before the organisation officially launched, we found ourselves on the receiving end of the smears and attacks that are all too familiar to cam-paigners everywhere. Some discovered my phone number and sent abusive text messages, while others trolled me and the rest of the team on social media sites. The har-assment from a small number of people was incessant, and highly stressful. I saw a very ugly side to politics early on. I received several threats of being referred to the GMC, our regulator, for my campaigning activities, so instead of returning to NHS work, I decided to work in Ireland as a doctor temporarily. The geographical distance and the remoteness of my location allowed me to compartmentalise the abuse to an extent, and to keep working. We all just soldiered on, the whole team. We had a clear cause and we stuck to it: to advocate for patients, staff and the future of the NHS.

The growth of EveryDoctor and the development of our network brought to light the true scale of many problems in the NHS. During one winter crisis, for example, we had a tip-off from a journalist about a lack of paediatric in-patient beds in one hospital. We reached out to our network of doctors to discover if the same thing was happening elsewhere, and were inundated with information coming back from NHS paediatric consultants. They were extremely concerned about the evolving situation. We gathered their testimony and fed this to a journalist at a national newspaper, who wrote it up to reveal what was happening and hold the government to account. We could see that our campaigning work was beginning to have an impact, so towards the end of 2019 we arranged meetings with a number of other journalists with a view to planning our next steps for larger-scale campaigns to raise public awareness about the problems occurring in NHS workplaces. We wanted to know how we could grow as an organisation, to achieve more.

Horrifyingly, that growth – our ability to speak to much wider audiences and effect change – happened sooner than any of us could have anticipated when the COVID-19 pandemic began in March 2020. Doctors within our network were watching closely, and when new information about the virus and its risks became available, they shared this throughout our network. The situation was evolving extremely quickly, and there was huge concern, even in those early days, that the UK government wasn't doing enough to safeguard both patients and NHS staff in many ways. It soon became apparent, for example, that many NHS workplaces didn't have enough Personal Protective Equipment for healthcare workers to wear to protect themselves or their patients.[10]

My husband was on a sabbatical from his central London teaching hospital at the time, but within a matter of days was asked to return to help run their intensive care unit, one of the largest in the UK. Ireland suddenly shut down all childcare facilities, as the virus began to spread like wildfire across the globe. I had been due to speak at a conference in the UK on behalf of EveryDoctor, but the event was cancelled at the last minute. Travel plans were up in the air, and things were changing hour by hour. We had no one to help us to look after the children, and so we couldn't both work clinically. We had a choice: remain in Ireland, or return to London to enable my husband to work as an ICU consultant. We opted for the second, just before the airports shut down. Luckily, the medical team I had been working with in Ireland was incredibly supportive of our need to be in London, and recognised that I couldn't easily continue my clinical work. We moved back into our one-bedroom flat with our two tiny children, which was difficult because it had no outdoor space, and the playground nearby was soon locked shut like almost everything else. However, despite everything, there was a strange comfort in coming home.

The EveryDoctor community, rapidly growing at this point, pulled together in the face of the crisis. The information sharing and collective support between doctors was fast-flowing, and themes began to emerge within their concerns. It became apparent that the UK was unprepared in several key ways, and that frontline healthcare workers themselves were insufficiently unprotected from coronavirus, which we realised would impact on the workers themselves and also on their patients. Frontline workers were tragically becoming unwell as a result, and some were dying.[11] The medical community was struggling to obtain answers from the government and from central bodies responsible for keeping staff and patients safe. It was clear that a campaign was required to lobby for immediate protections for NHS workers. And so our network of doctors built that campaign, bringing over a hundred MPs on board and helping to secure vital protections for this vulnerable group.[12]

Doctors were working extremely long hours, going above and beyond for their patients, and yet many spent their limited time off advocating for patients and bringing crucial information into the public domain, often at great risk to themselves. The rules around doctors speaking up in the press, which had always been strict, tightened significantly. One major teaching hospital banned consultants from talking to the *Guardian* or the *Financial Times*, another conducted an aggressive witch-hunt to identify which doctor had provided a quote for the press. Our EveryDoctor members bravely spoke up again and again. We were bombarded by press outlets wanting to hear medical perspectives, and our members wrote opinion pieces for newspapers both in the UK and internationally, and provided comment for hundreds of written and broadcast pieces in between their gruelling shifts on the NHS frontline. Some of the doctors who felt compelled to speak were very senior, and were privy to information that wasn't being made public. We set up a system enabling a number of them to be interviewed by a trusted investigative journalist, and their audio interviews were then re-recorded by an actor to safeguard their identities.

We also set up weekly parliamentary briefings for politicians. We had realised that many politicians were struggling to access factual information about what was happening, and to properly understand the problems facing the NHS. So we instituted parliamentary meetings every Thursday, inviting every MP to hear from frontline doctors, who explained the issues. It was a crash course in parliamentary protocol, interactions with politicians and party politics. A small team of volunteers called round MP offices each week, asking them to attend the meetings, a strategy that proved highly effective, as numbers rose steadily to 20, 30, 40 MP attendees. For many politicians, it became a regular fixture in their diaries. Many spoke up and pushed for change in various ways, using their positions to influence policy and do everything they could.

We spoke regularly on the phone to various MPs to update them on particular aspects of the emerging crisis, and our team helped them to construct questions for Prime Minister's Questions, speeches for Parliament, letters to ministers. Our doctor members highlighted a number of emerging situations to politicians and the press; for example, the unsafe PPE being sent out to NHS workplaces, some of which was years out of date,[13] and in a number of cases was warped and broken. We spoke up about the deteriorating mental health of those working on the frontline, the trauma and the exhaustion, and many other disturbing aspects of this national emergency.

And between the weekly MP briefings and the endless round of media interviews, we tried to provide some support for our community, setting up a texting network between our members. Each of us would text a group of doctors regularly just to check in and provide emotional support. We leant on each other enormously during this time. It never felt enough; our community and so many others endured deep trauma. The government wholly failed to protect NHS workers during the pandemic or to properly support them to safely care for patients. It has left deep scars for UK doctors; I don't think they will ever forget how profoundly the government failed NHS staff and patients during that dreadful time. My husband worked all hours, often gone before 6am and back after midnight. From the windows of our flat every Thursday evening we'd hear the sound of applause as our local community clapped for the NHS. My husband looked numb when this happened. He looked numb all the time, dazed and ashen-faced.

Running our campaign during the pandemic taught me many things about campaigning, about the political landscape of the UK. It taught me that change can be effected when NHS workers and staff speak up together, and that despite various media campaigns in recent years splitting the two groups (accusing NHS staff of laziness or greed, or blaming patients, who are sometimes depicted as expecting too much from the service), ultimately NHS patients and staff want the same thing. We all want a functioning, safe, excellent health service in which staff are supported to do their jobs well, caring for patients.

I learned too that there are no bounds to the betrayal that some politicians are happy to stoop to in order to achieve their political goals. At the height of the pandemic, a time of great sacrifice for so many people, many politicians ignored plea after plea from struggling frontline workers, minimising concerns as their friends and colleagues died. Some politicians conducted press interviews and sent out reassuring emails about things they had no right to be reassuring anyone about. At times they deliberately misrepresented the truth, even when we were in the middle of a national crisis. Even when the only useful tools we had were transparency and honesty, the ability to work together, pool what we had and seek practical solutions to improve things for people as much as possible.

Political actions that take place as a process over a long period of time, contributed to by many people, can be difficult to analyse. It can be hard to attribute decision-making to one particular person or one particular moment. And because of this, many politicians have got away with wrongdoing involving the NHS for many decades now. Previous governments, governments that have now ended and that we can no longer hold to account for the decisions they enacted, took action that did not further the aims of the NHS or serve patients. Decisions to allow private providers to infiltrate the service. Decisions to build new hospitals not through funding them with public taxation, but by outsourcing the projects to the private sector and saddling the NHS with colossal debt as a result.

But actions during a crisis are more easy to pinpoint, and it was therefore incredibly illuminating to watch the government's response to the pandemic. We were able to scrutinise, day by day, the decisions made by Boris Johnson and Matt Hancock and others. We watched politicians receive thousands of emails highlighting concerns, and we watched what they did next. We watched who responded and we watched who ignored them. We watched the responses they sent to constituents and we watched closely to see who attended our weekly meetings to speak to frontline doctors, who then lobbied for vaccines for healthcare workers, or safe PPE, or death-in-service benefits for the healthcare workers who were dying, horrifyingly, in large numbers because of a lack of safe protections.

Most profoundly of all, the pandemic taught me about the energy that can propel a campaign from being a mere idea to prompting a government policy change in an extremely short period if enough people are pulling in the same direction and the media are engaged – energy that I hadn't really known existed until then. It highlighted the utter humanity of so many people who care deeply about the NHS and want to do something about it. This gave me, and gives me, so much hope about what we can demand, what we can change when we unite and push for those changes together.

Our network grew. We ventured onto Twitter, and Instagram; we grew a mailing list, and began to talk not only to doctors about what was happening, but to lots of people all over the UK: other healthcare workers, NHS supporters, campaigners, patients, relatives of patients. And as the major waves of the pandemic ebbed away and new issues came to the fore, our incredible network began to lobby against NHS privatisation and aired our concerns about the Health and Care Act 2022. We spoke up about the court case which we were bringing against the government, and then the outcome, and the need to hold politicians to account. We lobbied for medical graduates who had been left on a waiting list to be given jobs within the NHS, and secured these. Our network continues to grow, and as it does so, its collective power grows as well. We can effect change. We have proved that multiple times now. And that matters more than ever before.

As I write this book, in early 2023, the NHS is collapsing, just as many predicted it would, and it is doing so because of the machinations of politicians over some four decades. Between 1980 and 2010, many politicians took decisions that weakened the NHS. They introduced an internal marketplace, they loaded the service with outsourced debt, and they fragmented it into tiny parts, thousands of which have been outsourced and are run by non-NHS providers including private companies.

INTRODUCTION

And having weakened the service, politicians since 2010 have reduced budgets hugely, so that we entered the pandemic in what was already a very precarious situation, with over four million NHS patients on waiting lists. The pandemic then caused huge numbers of operations to be delayed and cancelled repeatedly, as well as severely affecting the provision of much specialist healthcare.

Those waiting lists continued to rise, month after month, beating the previous record of 'the longest NHS waiting lists ever recorded' again and again. Waiting times for ambulances and in A&E have lengthened dramatically, and hundreds of NHS staff are leaving the service every week, due to lack of support or the failure to pay them properly. And instead of listening to healthcare leaders, who spoke up repeatedly about what was happening and proposed sensible, rational solutions, politicians ignored them. Disgracefully, staff have been blamed for the problems. GPs, in particular, have borne the brunt of relentless scapegoating, criticism and abuse. They each look after two or three thousand people, sometimes more. If those people cannot easily access specialist treatment, they often get sicker. They require more time, more medications. Their health often deteriorates, their quality of life may decrease. Some may even develop mental health problems. And through all of this, a patient's GP is responsible for their care. This is an enormously stressful burden of responsibility. But GPs, instead of being supported in this situation, have been on the receiving end of attacks in the media and from politicians. They have been blamed for the problems, and have faced criticism for not seeing enough patients face to face. These attacks have been so extensive and so pervasive that they have caused many patients to become angry with their GP. It has led to a rise in patient abuse towards staff. I have heard many incidents of threatened violence, extensive verbal abuse, doors kicked in at GP surgeries. One GP was even attacked by a patient and left with a fractured skull.

This situation is appalling. Since the pandemic, pressures upon staff have escalated, and yet they are the ones blamed for problems. They often propose solutions, but these are ignored by the government. For a considerable time, the service has been going in one direction, and one direction only: towards wholesale collapse. And that collapse has now happened. An estimate put out by the Royal College of Emergency Medicine in early 2023 showed that up to five hundred patients a week were dying needlessly due to delays in urgent and emergency care. As I write this, there are reports from our network of patients falling and breaking their hips and calling for an ambulance that never comes; of elderly patients dialling 999 in an emergency only for the ambulance to take so long to arrive that the patient has died by the time it arrives. Patients are being administered life-saving treatment behind curtains held up by other staff, in busy waiting rooms. The situation is a humanitarian crisis.

And still, the politicians have failed to take proper responsibility for what has happened, and is happening. They refuse to recognise the situation as it is and respond in the strongest ways possible. They are failing to support the staff, to treat the situation as an emergency, to accept responsibility for the public. The NHS is collapsing, and it is not collapsing because of unavoidable circumstances, or because of an unexpected bout of flu or COVID-19, or because GPs are lazy, or because patients are turning up at A&E when they don't need to. The situation cannot be blamed on individuals who are seeking healthcare in vulnerable moments or on the overworked staff who are holding the service together as best they can. It is the culmination of political decisions that have taken place over the past 40 years, the results of which started slowly but are now rushing to their natural conclusion – the conclusion we witness all around us: the collapse of our public healthcare system.

This is a book I have felt compelled to write as a campaigner. The NHS belongs to the public, but ready access to comprehensive care is being taken away now. The government and their political opposition are proposing solutions to this crisis that simply will not solve it; their suggested measures do not tackle the deep problems within the NHS and instead promote more outsourcing, wastage, and the funnelling of public money into the private healthcare sector. This will not serve NHS patients or staff. Politicians have no mandate to continue along their current course, starving the public service of resources while lining the pockets of private company shareholders. Their betrayals have gone on for long enough. It is time to stop them in their tracks, unpick their damage and reimagine what we want from the NHS. If we want it to survive for another 75 years, we will need to fight for it, because its current trajectory is very advanced now. There won't be 75 more years unless there is a change of course; too many things have already been cut away, underfunded and privatised. If we want the NHS to survive as a public service, we are going to have to fight for it together.

1
THE PROMISE

The NHS is an extraordinary institution, one that has endured for 75 years. And sometimes, because various politicians have used the service as a political gambling chip, a rosette, a flag that they can shimmy up their own flagpole to signal their allegiance to 'the people', it can be easy to lose sight of the fact that it is not a favour bestowed upon us by the good grace of benevolent politicians, theirs to give or take away or shape as they choose, but instead a public service with clearly stated aims. It is a public service governed by three clear principles, which are stated within the NHS constitution on the UK government's own website.

These principles indicate that the NHS will provide equal care for all, based on a patient's clinical need, and provided for free at the point of delivery. Together, they represent the promise of the NHS: a promise made to every member of the public and one that explains why the NHS has become embedded within our society. For 75 years, we have relied upon it to care for us during our hour of need as well as some of the pivotal moments of our lives.

If you have been picked up by an NHS ambulance during an emergency or received care during an incredibly difficult time, perhaps for yourself or a loved one, you remember those moments. Key events that have shaped the person you are now may well have involved the NHS. When I worked as a junior doctor in A&E, one of my seniors said to us frequently, 'this is just another day at work for you. But for your patients, this is a moment they might remember forever.' And they were right. I remember clearly the times when I gave birth in an NHS maternity ward, received emergency care in an A&E department, visited a member of my family when they were extremely unwell and receiving world-class NHS treatment. I don't think it's in any way outlandish, then, to suggest that the NHS has become a part of our consciousness, our national identity. For 75 years, it has provided the backdrop to millions of lives.

There have been various articles written recently in the media, or statements from politicians, which bemoan 'mawkish'[1] attitudes towards the NHS, or the 'religious fervour'[2] with which the NHS is spoken about. But in my experience, as a medical student within the NHS and then as a doctor, a campaigner and a patient, the feelings engendered by the health service aren't mawkish. They aren't anything other than the felt effects of the power of a public service governed by these three core principles.

I entered medical school in 2004, and it was a time of great optimism within healthcare and the NHS. There was the feeling that things were improving: that new developments were occurring, waiting lists being driven down, new initiatives and research being invested in. There was a genuine energy in the way people spoke about the service, about its potential and the positive impact it was having on millions of people's lives. It felt like an absolute privilege to be studying within the NHS, and that sense of privilege stayed with me when I qualified and began working within the system.

The NHS has been set up so that the costs of the immediate delivery of care to a patient are not discussed. Clinicians are aware of the costs of delivering healthcare; for example, how much different blood tests cost to run, the cost of ordering an X-ray or the comparative cost of prescribing one drug or another. This is important because the NHS is a public service funded by taxes, and has never been awash with funds. And there are occasionally times when a patient requires a drug or treatment that is not provided by the NHS, often because it is new or extremely expensive. These situations lead to cost calculations and debates that often reach the public domain, and sometimes result in a re-evaluation of what needs to be provided by the NHS. But crucially, any such discussions happen outside of the interactions between an NHS patient and the staff members treating them. Clinical decision-making is solely based on what a patient needs. And this is extremely powerful. It places a patient and their care at the heart of all service delivery.

This system is one of the reasons why people value the NHS so highly. In many other countries, even before a patient has received any medical treatment, they have to prove that they can afford it (by sharing either their credit card or health insurance details). And even when a staff member is not tasked with directly checking a patient's ability to pay, the consideration of costs is still ever-present. If, for example, a patient is relying on their healthcare insurance to pay for their treatment, many will have a ceiling to the level of treatment they can gain access to. This means that as they are being assessed, the cost of various diagnostic tests or treatments will need to be calculated and considered to assess what can be afforded, and what cannot. Healthcare is extremely expensive. Treatment for severe illnesses can cost tens or even hundreds of thousands of pounds.

For many people, this is a devastating state of affairs; one in which huge numbers put off seeing their doctor until their symptoms become too severe to ignore, in the hope that things will improve on their own. They try home remedies, or take over-the-counter medications such as painkillers, in an attempt to stem symptoms of underlying conditions that require medical attention. Tragically, this means that for some diagnoses, the disease will be very advanced by the time the person accesses treatment, which may limit the options available to them. Some in such countries do seek healthcare when they become unwell, but the bills are so high that they often cripple them and their families financially. If you cannot access healthcare that fully meets your needs, your symptoms may worsen. You may require additional medications, some of which may be addictive, have serious side effects, or cause your health to deteriorate in other ways. An inability to access healthcare can devastate people's lives, the immeasurable stress destroying careers and contributing to family breakdowns, not to mention placing additional burdens of care on unpaid carers, which can widen inequality.

In the US, healthcare costs are the number-one cause of bankruptcy, because of their sheer scale.[3] These costs aren't always clear when a patient seeks help (depending on the diagnostic tests required, treatment, length of hospital stay, they can vary enormously and stack up fast), so, upon recovery, patients can suddenly find themselves inundated with unexpected medical bills, a considerable time after their actual treatment. This often leads to lengthy negotiations between a patient or their family and a healthcare provider in which costs are questioned and re-calculated, to establish the amount that must be paid. All of this is enormously stressful, particularly so when people are struggling, unwell, recovering, or even grieving the loss of a loved one who has died in hospital. The situation is terrible. When you compare it to the way the NHS is run, a healthcare system like that of the US seems incredibly inhumane; the cost of human health, and life, writ large in the starkest of terms on hospital bills.

The knowledge that everybody's health is valued, and that every person will be supported to optimise theirs, and be cared for should it start to fail, is therefore extremely powerful. The health of a nation, after all, has benefits far beyond the treatment of illness. It has impacts on the happiness of its people and even their productivity, which therefore impacts on a nation's economy. The provision of public healthcare across the UK provides a bedrock of support that has shaped our society for the past 75 years.

In accordance with the principles stipulated by the NHS constitution, the system within the NHS was built specifically to promote the provision of fair and equitable care to patients. If we take the example of a specialist NHS mental health team, staff members work within a team of other professionals. There will likely be a mixture of clinical skills within the team: doctors, psychologists, nurses, support workers and others. Each team shares a 'caseload' of patients: those who are currently receiving care. As well as providing ongoing care for these, the team will constantly receive referrals for new patients. The team will work through the new referrals as quickly as they can to ensure that waiting times are minimised. All of the patients who are waiting to be seen are placed on a waiting list based on the length of time since their referral, to ensure that those who have waited the longest are seen first. However if a new referral is received that indicates the patient is in an emergency situation, or that their condition has deteriorated significantly while waiting for an initial appointment, that patient immediately jumps the queue. At any time, a team must balance its resources effectively so that all patients under its care receive what they need.

Crucially, patients are prioritised depending on their clinical need, not their ability to pay. You cannot jump the queue within the NHS by paying more. This system, prioritising the sickest patients and offering them whatever they need based on their clinical condition, applies across all NHS services. The NHS is a series of interlinked facilities and teams operating all across the UK, providing hospital and community care for every medical speciality. The principle of fairness governs the way that the NHS runs across the entire country, and this system confers trust. It is collaborative, highly effective and keeps people safe, as long as the service is properly funded. In an Ipsos Mori poll conducted in August 2022, the public was asked, 'what makes us proud to be British?', and the NHS came out on top.[4] There is deep pride in how the NHS is set up and the way it delivers care.

But this system alone isn't enough to fulfil the three core principles governing the NHS. In order to provide care that is equal and comprehensive, meeting the needs of an entire population, the NHS should also be responsive to the changing needs of our population. Society isn't static; the demographics change, and our understanding of health and disease are ever-changing too. Purely looking at age demographics, things have changed enormously since the NHS began in 1948. Data from the Office of National Statistics (ONS) shows that within the first 70 years of the NHS's existence, male life expectancy increased from 65.9 years to 79.5 years, and that of females from 70.3 years to 83.1 years.[5] This is a huge lengthening of life expectancy (in part, due to the work of the NHS itself), and is something to be celebrated. But longer lives also create a significant change in the shape of our society and the healthcare needs of our population as a whole. Older people generally have more complex healthcare requirements, and in addition to the acute care they may need, in the form of A&E attendances and hospital admissions, a growing number of people are living with multiple chronic conditions requiring active management. This is progress, a result of people living longer. But it is also a challenge, requiring those making decisions about the NHS to respond in an agile way to best meet patient needs.

Beyond this demographic issue, there is the additional challenge of understanding patients' experiences within the system. Patients are not a homogeneous group; people have different experiences in accessing health-care, and there are significant structural barriers affecting many groups of patients that we are only just starting to understand. There is important work to be done, listening and learning from non-white patients, from people with disabilities, from people experiencing neuro-diversity, from trans people, from immigrants and other groups. The promise and principles of the NHS present a dynamic challenge to deliver good healthcare to every person. Its structures and processes must evolve to better meet patients' needs. The NHS promise will never be fulfilled if it's framed as a static goal; a set number of hospitals, GP surgeries and members of staff, for example. It should be an ever-evolving project, assessing where those healthcare facilities are, how healthcare is being delivered, the involvement of technology, the diversity in representation within the leadership that makes decisions, and numerous other factors.

And beyond all of this is the inevitable consideration of costs. Public healthcare doesn't exist in a vacuum; it's sensitive to the costs of drugs and equipment, to infla-tion, and to staff salaries. The costs of running a healthcare service increase every year[6] even if the provision of healthcare remains static. And healthcare itself doesn't remain static; our evidence base grows, new developments occur, pioneering research is carried out. These bring new medicines, new operations, new diagnostic procedures. We have changing expectations as a population about what healthcare can and should provide for us. We now employ ten times as many doctors as we did in 1948.[7] Many of our medical specialities since then have changed so much as to be unrecognisable, in terms of what is available to help patients. Progress has been endless, whether in the approach to and treatment of mental illness, the development and use of antibiotics, surgical advances, emergency care, or the development of entirely new medical specialities including intensive care medicine. In order to fulfil the promise of the NHS, governments should be mindful of the priorities of the electorate and of delivering on those. If, as looks to be the case, the public wants our public healthcare service to be prioritised within a given government's spending, this should be adhered to.

The NHS project, so boldly started 75 years ago with a promise to deliver equal, comprehensive care free to all at the point of need, is extremely ambitious and extremely challenging. If politicians, any group of politicians at any time, hope to honour the promise made in the NHS constitution, then the work involved is significant. Delivering on its principles requires a significant commitment from whichever government is in charge at a given time, because the government sets the NHS budget. The government also has the ability to pass Bills that can reform the NHS and change its shape, structure and function. And so, despite NHS principles having remained the same for 75 years, the quality of the service and the delivery of its aims have been highly dependent on the degree of commitment that politicians have to it, and this situation will continue.

The NHS exists in the first place because a huge number of people in the middle of the twentieth century willed it into being. Conversations about the structure of society, and our collective responsibilities towards one another, are as old as civilisation itself. But during the early part of the twentieth century, these conversations became more prominent, and a sequence of events converged that resulted in the founding of the NHS. Following the Industrial Revolution, the great migration to cities and the expansion of the industrial workforce within Britain, many people started to wonder if our society should be rebuilt in a more egalitarian manner. The organisation of the industrial workforce was beneficial to those creating profit, who ascribed value to individuals based on the measurable output of their work. But this organisation of their labour began to benefit the workers too; it brought them together as effective units with collective power.

New, powerful ideas developed widespread support: about the importance of workers' rights, about providing support for those vulnerable people within our society who couldn't work, about the need for the state to step in and help such individuals instead of relying on the philanthropy of wealthy individuals. As part of these broad conversations, ideas and plans for a public healthcare system were debated rigorously in the years leading up to the Second World War. However there was opposition from many groups and individuals, some of whom were ideologically opposed to the concept, and others who struggled to understand how a public healthcare system could be built and run efficiently and sustainably.

It was the shared experiences of the war itself – the cohesion, the mutual dependency, the horror and the national trauma – that eventually propelled the NHS into being. Issues that might previously have felt academic or theoretical had become a reality. Our society had been forced together in order to survive together. Amid the trauma, an idea gained mass acceptance: that a good society takes responsibility for the care of every individual. A report called the Beveridge Report was published in 1942, which contained a plan for widespread social reform including a public health system. The report proved extremely popular with the public; more than 600,000 copies had been sold by February 1944.[8] The plans outlined within it provided architecture for powerful ideas of social change that were taking hold, and allowed people to imagine society functioning in a different way. The Labour Party paid close attention to these changing ideas. When their leader, Clement Attlee, campaigned to become Prime Minister in 1945, proposals within the Beveridge Report were hugely influential in shaping the policies of his General Election manifesto. He appealed to the public with a hopeful vision of social change, campaigning with the powerful message: 'Let Us Face the Future'. He won a landslide victory, in one of the largest vote swings of the twentieth century.[9]

The huge majority commanded in the House of Commons by the Labour Party enabled them to enact enormous changes over the next few years. This extraordinary period in British politics saw the rise of the welfare state and the implementation of National Insurance. National pensions were put into place, along with unemployment benefits and sickness benefits. Workers' rights were properly considered and improved, and a whole array of key industries were nationalised: coal mining, the steel industry, electricity and gas, the canals, the haulage industry. The changes were monumental, and the founding of the National Health Service was central to all of them. The NHS embodied and actively demonstrated the value that was being placed on the health of every single individual within our society.

Prior to the formation of the NHS, industrial workers in Britain did have some healthcare provision. This had been brought in with the National Insurance Act 1911,[10] in the form of a healthcare insurance scheme. The scheme had been revolutionary at the time, supporting workers through giving them access to sick leave and to medical attention from doctors, and it was paid for through contributions made by the workers, their employers and the government. However, the scheme only applied to wage-earners; their families and those not working were not covered. This system clearly signalled that those who were economically active were more deserving in terms of their health outcomes, which disregarded the needs of many of the most vulnerable people within society. Therefore, when the NHS began in July 1948, it was offering something radical. It was the first system of its kind anywhere in the world seeking to provide healthcare for every citizen, irrespective of their 'economic value'.

The NHS is not a single organisation spanning the UK; it actually comprises four separate healthcare systems: NHS England, NHS Wales, NHS Scotland and Health and Social Care (HSC) – the name given to the merger of the NHS with the social care system in 1973 – in Northern Ireland. The devolution occurred in a stepwise manner, beginning in 1948 at the inception of the NHS. The National Health Service Act of 1948 brought hospitals that had been run by local authorities into public ownership within both England and Wales, and similar Acts were passed concerning Scotland and Northern Ireland soon after this. The healthcare systems of the last two were managed between 1948 and 1999 by government departments: the Scotland Office and the Northern Ireland Office. Separate legislation was passed in 1969 that separated the Welsh NHS from the English one, putting the governance of the Welsh NHS under the Welsh Office of government. And in 1999, health became a devolved matter, responsibility for the healthcare systems being transferred to the Welsh Senedd, the Northern Ireland Assembly, and the Scottish Parliament.[11]

The NHS in each nation is underpinned by the same three principles: that the service meets every person's needs, that the care provided is free at the point of delivery, and that it is provided on the basis of clinical need, not on a person's ability to pay. However, the devolution of healthcare has allowed each nation to focus on the healthcare priorities of its own citizens.

The four nations' healthcare systems used to function quite similarly in their structure and design. But because there are now four separate healthcare systems, and the politicians in charge of the NHS in each nation have power over introducing new legislation and reforms, there are significant differences between them. The policies of political leaders in each nation have heavily influenced the development of their respective health services over the past few decades. And they have had a big impact. NHS prescriptions, for example, are free for all patients in Wales, Scotland and Northern Ireland, but only free in England if a patient fulfils certain criteria. There are differences that affect NHS staff as well as patients. For instance, I know of many doctors who chose to move to Scotland from England in the mid-2010s, because junior doctors in Scotland didn't have a contract imposed upon them in 2016 that disproportionately impacts on women.[12]

The NHS in England has also been infiltrated much more heavily by privatisation.[13] While none of the devolved nations are free from its creeping influence, the landscape is much more advanced and entrenched in England due to successive legislative changes made over the past few decades. For this reason, I am focusing on the NHS in England within this book. The state of the service should serve as a cautionary tale.

I spend a lot of my time campaigning against NHS privatisation, and one of the common questions that comes up when I am speaking to people about the changes to the NHS over time is 'Why would politicians want to privatise the NHS in the first place?' To answer this question, it's best to go back to the NHS principles and examine the political thinking behind the formation of the service. The NHS model of healthcare is based on tenets of collectivism and of taking responsibility as a society for the health of everyone, to the benefit of all. These are, in essence, socialist principles. Many of the governments we have had since the NHS's inception 75 years ago would probably not voluntarily choose to run a fully publicly owned, publicly run health service. Interestingly, many members of the public who support the NHS are not socialists themselves, but they value our public healthcare system highly and want it to continue following the same precepts with which it was initially constructed. And so we have a situation whereby the majority of the public wants the NHS to continue, and has not been publicly consulted on introducing privatisation into the service, yet many of our governments have taken successive steps to do exactly this.

Over the past 40 years, government ministers have made incremental changes to the structure of the service that have opened up the NHS to privatisation and external providers in many different ways. Starting in the 1980s, they created an internal NHS marketplace that forced NHS facilities to compete with one another. They also engaged in a huge number of private finance initiative (PFI) contracts that outsourced the building and maintenance of NHS facilities to private companies, thereby burdening the NHS with enormous debt and cripplingly expensive maintenance contracts with private providers. They introduced outsourcing of NHS services, which means that thousands are now run by external providers including private companies. And parts of the service are currently being sold off to private interests, including one instance recently of a large number of GP surgeries being sold to a healthcare insurance company.

Each of these changes over the past 40 years has, for two reasons, interfered with the NHS's ability to fulfil its principles and provide equal, comprehensive care for all. First, because of the disruption of the very architecture of the system. Making these changes within the NHS's structure has fragmented the system and damaged relationships between the services and, on an individual level, between staff and patients. And second, because in the pursuit of corporatisation within the service, policy makers have committed their attention to melding the service into a new shape, instead of devoting their energies towards furthering the three principles, expanding and evolving the NHS project.

But there have been times during the past 40 years when, despite all of these negative factors, the full scale of the damage caused by politicians' decisions has been masked because of the sheer scale of investment into the NHS. During the Blair years, for example, the largest expansion of PFI projects took place. Huge hospital projects were taken on, paid for and managed by private companies and then leased back to the NHS at great expense (which we are still paying for, billions of pounds of public money spent every single year[14]). But Blair's government also made record-breaking investments into the NHS[15] that drove down waiting lists and invested enormously in the service. There were fissures forming below the surface, destabilising the integrity of the

NHS's structure. But these were papered over with money; lots and lots of money.

Over the past decade and a bit, we have finally seen the true extent of the damage done by multiple governments over the past 40 years. And this is because, in addition to accelerating the privatisation of the service in a multitude of ways, successive governments since David Cameron's narrow 2010 election victory and subsequent coalition with the Lib Dems have starved the NHS of its funding,[16] cut hospital bed numbers,[17] instigated long-standing NHS staff pay freezes,[18] cut the student nurse bursary[19] that supported nurses through their studies (and then restarted it again, after much pressure from campaigners and the public[20]). They have failed to listen to repeated warnings from healthcare leaders, campaigners and the public about the long-term impact of their decisions; both these and others. You can't cut things back forever and expect the service to remain the same, expect the staff to keep absorbing more and more. There's a tipping point. Over time, the situation becomes intolerable, and things break. People's morale, the level of care that can be offered. The capacity of the healthcare facilities, which becomes overwhelmed (we currently, for example, have an unmet maintenance bill for building repairs in the NHS in England of £9 billion.[21] Some much-needed repairs have been shelved even though they've been judged a significant safety risk for staff and patients).

The problems built up as we got towards the end of the 2010s. The paper applied by New Labour peeled away, revealing the deepening cracks within the service.

Staff morale was dwindling fast after a decade of cutbacks and squeezes. Patient safety problems started to emerge, at first as isolated incidents during the busiest times of the year (the so-called 'winter crises' that became an annual occurrence from around 2013 onwards), and then at other busy times such as long bank holiday weekends when the service struggled with skeleton staff numbers. Doctors began to dread public holidays because we knew the stress they would entail; the pressure the service would be under and the impact on our patients. Everyone became stretched beyond capacity, and understaffing became a significant problem within the service.

For some time before long waiting lists and over-stretched A&E departments began making the headlines, pressures began building up for staff within the service. There were increasing instances of NHS doctors being expected to do the jobs of two or three. When doctors are placed in a position like this (because of staff absences and a failure to find anyone else to fill the slot) it's a stressful experience. Teams of doctors who are 'on-call' within each medical speciality work in a coordinated fashion to receive information about new patients, or patients requiring urgent attention within the hospital. This information is disseminated between team members, who then assess and treat patients in a safe and organised fashion. Because of the way healthcare facilities are laid out, the team will likely be covering several clinical areas at any given time. This requires each member of the team to carry a device through which they can be contacted (often a pager, or sometimes a mobile phone).

Information flows up the chain to the most senior doctor, and down the chain to the most junior. It is a system that has been developed to ensure optimal safety for patients.

If the team is missing one of its doctors, their device still needs to be carried by someone in the team, because they are the point of contact that other staff members use (for example, A&E staff referring a new patient, queries coming in from NHS facilities in the community, nurses on hospital wards who require assistance with a patient, the hospital switchboard informing the team about an emergency somewhere in the hospital requiring immediate attention). And so one of the remaining team members has to carry two devices.

This places the system under immediate pressure. As the calls come in with tasks requiring attention, the doctor receiving that information has to either make a further call, asking another team member to take action, or add the task to their own list. But any doctor doing the job of several people can quickly become swamped, with calls coming in faster than the tasks can be allocated or completed. Things quickly become fraught, and the situation can be extremely stressful. In situations like this, doctors run on adrenaline. There's barely time to eat or drink, or even to go to the loo. Such a state of affairs was once rare; notable. But over time, occurrences like these became more and more common, and if one team found itself in this position, the likelihood was that other teams in the hospital were facing something similar. The result has been stressed-out, over-stretched doctors calling other stressed-out, over-stretched doctors within the same hospital, to refer a patient, share information, or attempt to solve a problem in a system where the pressure never lets up. I've been in this situation many times. At the end of a day like this you feel exhausted, wrung out, hollow, and you are full of anxiety about whether you missed anything, rushed anything, failed to complete important tasks that could impact on someone's health.

Staffing gaps began long before the pandemic occurred. There were many instances where staffing shortages occurred, and because the doctors 'coped', little effort would be put into recruiting staff into the team gaps that created these situations. Gradually, it became the norm to take on the work that traditionally would have been managed by multiple doctors. This affected doctors a lot, and it affected other staff groups too, who faced different but equally stressful pressures. If you come home from work wrung out, you have little energy to engage with your family or friends. It can affect lots of things; it can be isolating and can start to affect your relationships.

We lost a huge number of experienced NHS clinicians during these years, towards the end of the 2010s. They chose to move abroad, or change careers, or retire early because of the pressures and stress they had to shoulder within an under-resourced system. I remember writing the information for EveryDoctor's website when we were planning our launch at the end of 2018. Even then, we were describing these pressures upon staff, the exodus of experienced professionals, the stress this was loading upon the remaining doctors and the impact it was having on patients.

The winter crises that received brief, intense media attention each year should have served as the canary in the mine, attracting the attention of the government and prompting the provision of resources to prevent the situation from continuing, and worsening. The staffing problems should have necessitated a response, particularly when evidence of low morale and an exodus of staff became apparent. The Chief Executive of the British Red Cross, after all, described the situation facing the NHS as a 'humanitarian crisis'[22] back in January 2017. There were deep-seated problems even then. And yet this didn't happen; there was no moment of reflection from the government, no re-evaluation of their plan for NHS budgeting or meaningful provision of staff support. And so the NHS entered the COVID-19 pandemic ill-equipped for the greatest public health challenge since its inception; with a depleted, exhausted workforce, and over four million patients on NHS waiting lists in England alone.[23]

In order to create capacity to care for patients who were extremely unwell with COVID-19, a lot of the planned elective procedures (non-emergency operations, for example, and outpatient appointments) were delayed or cancelled, sometimes multiple times.[24] Many staff were relocated from their usual workplaces to look after COVID-19 patients, often working beyond their professional experience, forced to step up at a time of crisis. This was necessary at the start of the pandemic, and despite the enormous pressure upon themselves, often involving a change in their working arrangements (or even their living arrangements), I didn't hear a single doctor complain about this. The stoicism was remarkable. I was running EveryDoctor full-time by this point, and spent much of my time corresponding with the doctors within our network. I was in regular contact with one of our members who is a surgeon, and who had decided to live away from his heavily pregnant wife because he felt compelled to be as available as possible to the patients in his hospital. There were many, many sacrifices like this among NHS staff members, and many instances of extraordinary stress absorbed by staff members.

The staff desperately required support to help them with the pressures they were experiencing, but any support given by the government seemed to be offered reluctantly, or not at all. The government eventually put 40 mental health hubs in place for staff in England,[25] but did so only after enormous campaigning efforts had made clear the dire need for these. Those efforts shouldn't have been necessary; the impact the pandemic had and continues to have on staff was obvious.[26] When vaccines became available, GPs in England were asked to set up many of the first vaccine centres at extremely short notice, and many doctors within our network pulled this off, working round the clock to ensure the safe set-up of these important facilities.[27] Frontline healthcare staff weren't prioritised for first-dose vaccines (again, not until enormous campaigning efforts pushed the government into action).[28] Staff were continually required to step up and give more, endure more sacrifice and hardship, and for many this was extremely difficult. I don't think there's been a proper reckoning of the experiences staff went through during that incredibly demanding time.

Of course, we should not underestimate the pressure the government would have been under during that time. Presumably they were being pulled in all directions. A huge number of people would have been placing demands on their desks. But I have to say that, having campaigned throughout the pandemic on many issues requiring immediate government attention – the lack of PPE, pay for temporary staff members who became sick, death-in-service benefits for many staff members, provision of urgent vaccines for frontline health and social workers – it didn't feel as if the government was on the front foot. Again and again, large groups of doctors and others asked the government to pay attention to situations that would safeguard lives, and were ignored or dismissed, the government only finally being pushed into action when the sheer number of people pushing for change forced it into a U-turn because of the political capital at stake.

And when, eventually, the major waves of the pandemic tailed off, the NHS was in a terrible state. We had entered the pandemic with over four million patients waiting for treatment.[29] At the time of writing, there are 7.2 million patients on waiting lists in England.[30] The numbers didn't suddenly spike from four to seven million. They went up month after month, and as the numbers have increased, they've been accompanied by lengthening waiting times in A&E[31] and for ambulances.[32] The government was repeatedly warned about the deteriorating situation, by campaigning organisations, trade unions, charities and Royal Colleges. For our part, EveryDoctor had the dates set into our calendar of when, every month, the NHS statistics in England would be announced. And every month we would discuss what was happening with the network of people we spoke to online. We would do our best to communicate the risks, to highlight the severity of the problems, to provide a platform for the concerns of frontline NHS doctors and the patient safety problems that were occurring. Month after month after month. Warning the public about what was happening. Warning about what would happen next. Organisations that traditionally have stayed pretty apolitical, medical organisations whose leaders had told me when we launched EveryDoctor that they could not risk being too 'strong' in their messaging about the government's actions, started being extremely explicit and critical in their public statements. They had no choice. It has become ever more evident since the summer of 2021 what was going to happen to the NHS. The situation was moving in one direction; towards full-blown collapse.

And that, as stated in the Introduction, has now happened. As I write this, in early 2023, the pressure at all levels of the health service is so enormous that the system is no longer holding together. Patients who need healthcare urgently, in emergencies, are often receiving no care at all. Many are dying while they wait. The pressures extend from community services like GP practices, all the way through the system. GPs usually assess people with new symptoms, treat acute illnesses, manage people's chronic diseases, and refer patients for specialist input where required. But because the burden of illness is so great within our communities now, GPs' time has become increasingly taken up with patients who are deteriorating while awaiting specialist input. They are providing urgent care and managing complex clinical decision-making for an increasingly sick group of patients, and meanwhile other people are unable to access a GP for routine appointments and check-ups. The pressure upon GPs at the moment is unbelievable, and mounting.

For patients who are unwell enough to need A&E treatment, ambulance waits are terrifyingly long. Every second counts when a patient is experiencing a clinical emergency. Ambulances attending life-threatening emergencies are taking far longer than the recommended waiting time to arrive. For patients with a stroke, severe burns or chest pain, at the time of writing the latest stats show an average wait of 93 minutes for an ambulance in England.[33] Through the network of doctors that EveryDoctor speaks to every day, we are hearing about patients who telephone for an ambulance that simply never arrives. Disturbing stories of patients eventually turning up at a GP practice many hours or even days later, having had a severe fall or breathlessness or chest pain. People who are trying to access healthcare and when they call, no one comes.

And for the patients who do reach A&E, the situations there are no better. In some cases, they're worse. Elderly patients waiting for 24 or 36 hours on seats in emergency waiting rooms, because there is no clinical area in which to treat them. Patients cared for in cupboards. Juggling plugs between patients requiring intravenous pump medications, because there aren't enough to go around. Hospital beds are being removed from the allocated spaces in the 'majors' areas of A&E departments to make way for six people sitting on chairs in each cubicle instead. One NHS consultant told me recently about a situation where an elderly person with a diagnosed stroke had had to sit for more than 24 hours on a waiting room chair. And this wasn't an isolated incident; the consultant described the overcrowding that was regularly forcing patients into situations like this. I've heard similar things from doctors all over the UK, who are horrified about the conditions their patients are enduring. So many instances of people waiting interminably, uncomfortably, without dignity, lacking the care they need. The care the staff are so desperately trying to provide. The care that patients deserve.

And meanwhile on hospital wards, staff battle day after day trying to care for patients as best they can, but frequently missing patients' medication doses because of the understaffing and the extraordinary pressures. Patients are discharging themselves, or their relatives (sometimes even babies, who are extremely unwell with conditions like sepsis) because they are so aghast at the conditions in the hospital and feel that they or their loved one is receiving care that is so substandard as to be pointless, and that they'd be better off at home. There are places where the staffing levels are so low now that patients' families are being asked to step in and provide care themselves in shifts. I spoke to one person recently who said her mum had been in hospital recently, desperately unwell with a rare form of cancer. She was being cared for in an intensive care unit, and required both chemotherapy and non-invasive ventilation. But because of the short staffing on her mum's ward, nursing staff without the correct intensive care training had been moved from other parts of the hospital to plug staffing gaps. The lady I spoke to described that on many occasions, none of the nursing staff on the ward knew how to work the non-invasive ventilation equipment properly, and as a desperate measure she had learned herself how to manage the equipment in some rudimentary fashion. Horrifyingly, on one occasion her mum's chemotherapy treatment was even paused, because none of the staff were confident about administering the drugs.

There is overcrowding everywhere, with stories of extra hospital beds being parked in the middle of six-bedded bays, with no curtains surrounding a bed-space for privacy. There are wards where beds are being jammed against emergency exits, because there is simply nowhere else to put them. This is a potential hazard, and some of these hospital beds don't have access to the things a patient might need, such as an oxygen supply. It is appalling, it is inhumane.

The social care crisis, which has been escalating for many years and which the current government has claimed on various occasions it will fix,[34] is extraordinarily bad. Carers aren't paid enough, there are staffing problems and capacity problems, and it's causing a situation in which huge numbers of patients are ready to be discharged from hospital but cannot leave. In an article in the *Guardian* published in November 2022,[35] it was revealed that in some NHS hospitals in England up to one in three patients was awaiting discharge in this way.

And for the staff, those pressures that I experienced in 2018, those bad days running on adrenaline, feeling stressed and fraught, must be looked back upon with relative fondness. Things are so much worse now. I receive information from doctors in our network who have been updating me regularly for several years about what's been happening where they are. I hear about what they're experiencing, their fears for their patients, their abject horror and sorrow, and the weight of their worries is often palpable through their words. Countless doctors and healthcare staff are showing extraordinary courage at the moment, repeatedly going the extra mile on behalf of their patients within a service that is collapsing all around them.

And aside from the minute-to-minute, day-to-day experiences in GP surgeries, A&E departments and hospital wards, there is the impact these experiences have on patients and relatives. These experiences won't easily be forgotten. They will stay, imprinted upon the memories of people who have been failed. Failed at the very time they required support. Failed in their most vulnerable moments. Failed because the operation was cancelled, again, or the treatment in A&E was administered too late. Failed because there wasn't a bed, or an appointment, or a plug, or someone who knew how to turn on the machine or give out the drugs. The NHS is broken, now.

The public can no longer rely on the promise of providing equitable, comprehensive care that is free at the point of use. And despite the emotionality of the situation, the deep, searing outrage at witnessing the collapse of something that was once whole and has been wilfully dismantled at the cost of human life, we must approach this situation in rational terms, removing emotion from the equation.

When governments take on the custodianship of the NHS, they are not agreeing to run a public health system with unspecified aims. They are taking on the custodianship of a public service that the public has consistently voiced support for. For example, the King's Fund conducted a project in 2017 as the NHS approached its seventieth birthday. They found 'around 90 per cent of people support the founding principles of the NHS, indicating that these principles are just as relevant today as when the NHS was established'.[36] Politicians over the past four decades have broken the NHS, broken its promise, and they have done so without a mandate. We must examine what has happened, in order to fight for its restoration.

2

THE BETRAYAL

The NHS is collapsing all around us, and patients are coming to harm. And the question that a lot of people are asking at the moment is 'why'? Why are so many people coming to harm? Why has this been allowed to happen? Why have things got so bad? And the answer, in a nutshell, is that successive governments have been tasked with running the NHS according to the principles written within its constitution, and they have failed to adhere to these principles. This catastrophe hasn't just been caused by the current politicians, but by those who have come before them as well. Politicians have power over decisions that impact on the running of the NHS; for example, the budgets made available to it. And politicians also make decisions concerning the long-term trajectory of the health service; they draw up legislation and push this through Parliament to make changes in the way that it is structured and functions.

Because there is a clearly stated NHS constitution that sets out the aims of our public healthcare system, our politicians should be governed and directed in their decision making by these objectives: of delivering a healthcare service that provides comprehensive care, equitable care, and care that is free at the point of access to everyone. The principles should be front and centre at all times, and they should form a mission statement, a manifesto, holding the government accountable and keeping the project on track. But this has not been the case. Politicians have been able, over the NHS's long tenure, to make decisions that deviate enormously from its founding principles. And a lot of decisions, large and small, over the years, have led to where we are today. The structure of the service has been fragmented enormously, its resources have been starved, and funding has been cut. All of this has led to the collapse of the NHS.

There are various myths that circulate about the NHS. One of the most pervasive and inaccurate is the idea that NHS staff are in control of the service, and that it is within their power to improve things. Many politicians are happy to propagate this myth, and numerous media outlets contribute to this misunderstanding too. But it simply isn't true; politicians set the agenda. NHS staff are tasked with managing the service and keeping patients safe within it, but they don't determine the budgets. They don't determine how many beds there are or how well supported and well paid the staff are. They aren't responsible for the poor IT systems and the over-crowding and the long waiting lists. They're managing as best as they can with the resources they're given. Given by the government.

Let's imagine for a moment that the NHS is a very old car, 75 years old, and the car needs to keep running. It has parts that are difficult to change (as do hospitals, many of which are extremely old buildings), and it has parts that are inefficient (again paralleled in hospitals, where significant energy wastage means they are often draughty, leaky and cold). It's very expensive to change those old parts, because to do so would cost a lot of money, but keeping them going is problematic too. There's lots of deliberation about whether the parts should be replaced. But on top of those considerations, the car is also driving down a bumpy road, full of twists and turns. Because the patient population is changing, technology is changing, medicine is changing, and people's expectations about the car itself are changing.

Politicians are tasked with deciding whether to replace the parts, sort the tyres out, fix the roof when it's leaking, and refill the petrol when it's running low. Some of our politicians, the custodians of this car, have taken their role pretty seriously when it's been their turn during the past 75 years. But others have not. Some have chosen not to replace the things that needed replacing, which has led to efficiency failures and safety problems. Others have chosen to take the car to a garage and install an entirely new engineering system, which hasn't suited either the car or the passengers, but has made someone some money. And the canniest of all have painted over the cracks on the exterior while simultaneously ripping out the engine.

Let's imagine that the NHS doctors and nurses are the drivers of the car, and the patients are the passengers. The drivers have had very little say in what happens to the car; they've just had to keep driving it, attempting to keep it in the right lane, chugging along safely. Meanwhile, the passengers are susceptible to whatever problems the car develops. If politicians haven't bothered sorting out the suspension, the patients are bumped around. If they haven't filled up the fuel tank, the car stops in the middle of the road and the passengers don't get to where they need to go. Crucially, the people in the driving seat are not actually in the driving seat at all. The politicians are sitting there instead. And at 75 years old, the NHS is an amalgamation of the decisions they have made. Our public healthcare system has therefore been vulnerable to their decision-making; to their whims, their personal interests, and whichever external influences they are vulnerable to at any given time.

Ultimately, the amalgamation of those decisions has led to disaster. We see the evidence all around us. If we want to understand why the NHS is in its current state, why this situation has been able to occur, it is important to consider the factors influencing politicians' decision-making. To consider what is leading them to make decisions that don't follow the NHS aims, don't place patients front and centre, and don't keep that car running safely. And the most obvious place to start is politicians' personal political ideologies. After all, one would expect that they would be largely motivated by their own beliefs about the provision of a public healthcare system.

It makes sense to start at the top, so let's consider the ideology of our Prime Minister, Rishi Sunak. Sunak has openly said in recent months that people cannot expect the state to 'fix every problem'.[1] He has also put forward proposals to start charging NHS patients for missed GP appointments (the proposal has since been dropped, when Sunak declared that it was 'not the right time'[2] for this initiative to be started). Both of these things are a huge red flag, because Sunak, as leader, is ultimately tasked with managing the resourcing of the NHS, along with other public services.

We learned about Sunak's political ideology during the chaotic summer months of 2022 following the demise of Boris Johnson's premiership. Sunak was locked in a head-to-head bid for the leadership of the Conservative Party (and thus to become Prime Minister) against his political rival Liz Truss. During this period – a frantic campaign that saw hastily put-together hustings across the UK, and Sunak preparing campaign packs for journalists that included 'Ready for Rishi' sunscreen and miniature cans of sprite[3] – both politicians were very vocal in their support of 'Thatcherism'.[4] They competed in putting forward very similar political rhetoric about minimising state involvement in citizens' lives, lowering taxes, and pulling back from the provisions of the welfare state.

To many people watching these campaigns unfold, the political messaging felt very jarring, amid a cost-of-living crisis and energy crisis in which many members of the public were really struggling to get by. A lot of people felt that the government should be providing more support for the public, not less. Sunak lost the bid for the leadership, but ended up as Prime Minister anyway, following an extraordinary few weeks in which Liz Truss won the contest, took the helm and swiftly tanked the UK economy. Sunak has only been in position for a few months, and it remains to be seen how readily he applies his self-proclaimed Thatcherite mentality to the NHS. So far, it's not looking good. He is presiding over the most severe crisis within the NHS's history, and isn't approaching the situation with the urgency one might expect, given that at the time of writing, it has been estimated that up to five hundred people are needlessly dying every single week[5] because of an inability to access the care they need.

The ideologies of those politicians most closely involved with the NHS have always attracted a great deal of curiosity, specifically because of the power that senior politicians have over the health service and its direction of travel. As our Health Secretary between 2010 and 2017, the longest-serving Health Secretary we have ever had, Jeremy Hunt has been the recipient of a great deal of such curiosity. Many commentators have drawn attention to Hunt's involvement in writing a 2005 policy book entitled *Direct Democracy: An Agenda for a New Model Party*,[6] which comprised the writings of a group of Conservative MPs, including Hunt. The book contained a chapter that provided a plan to replace the NHS with a health insurance system, involving the private sector. Hunt has since attempted to distance himself from this rhetoric, claiming that he did not write the chapter about the NHS. However, the book was presented as a whole, without denoting the authors of each chapter, and Hunt was declared to be one of the authors of the book.

As a keen observer of Hunt's actions for almost a decade now, I find his ideology difficult to ascertain. He was Health Secretary during a period that saw unfair contracts being imposed upon junior doctors, the stopping of student-nurse bursaries, significant staff pay freezes and bed cuts. But since leaving his post as Health Secretary, he has been a key advocate for patient safety and has made some extremely helpful suggestions about the future direction of the service. Frankly, many of the doctors I speak to feel perplexed about this. Hunt seemed to have successfully rebranded himself as an advocate of the NHS by the time he became Chancellor of the Exchequer in autumn 2022 (an extraordinary feat, given the low opinions many doctors had held about him previously). But he is yet to take action on the NHS pensions crisis – an issue he is well aware of and has spoken publicly about – which is pushing some senior doctors into cutting their hours because of the outlandish tax they are being charged on their pension contributions (in many cases, more than 100 per cent to take on extra shifts,[7] meaning they are effectively paying to go to work during the worst NHS crisis we have ever experienced).

Of course, any information willingly offered by a politician about their beliefs and priorities must be received with a degree of scepticism. Margaret Thatcher, key architect of NHS privatisation, was very careful to keep her cards close to her chest. Thirty-five years ago, Thatcher set up a working group to discuss reforming the NHS. A recent biography claims that 'the Prime Minister never ceased to worry that the NHS had the potential to destroy her politically and electorally', and apparently she was so concerned about public backlash to her plans that she 'had acted as the document's editor removing words which struck the wrong tone like "customers" and "competition" and replacing or adding more empathetic language'.[8] It was Thatcher and her government who began the long trajectory that has led us to a situation where thousands of NHS services in England are now run by external providers including private companies.

It's natural to be curious about the ideologies of our politicians, and with so many people struggling at the moment, during a tumultuous time within British politics and for our society in general, it can be tempting to think that if we could only find politicians whose personal ideologies aligned with the provision of a well-resourced welfare state, the public would benefit from this. But unfortunately, the issues are much more complicated than this. Personal political ideologies are only one piece of the puzzle.

I have noticed during the time that I have campaigned on issues relating to the NHS, that the engagement we receive from MPs changes significantly over time. Political parties create their own objectives and long-term goals and messaging, and this can sometimes hamper a politician's ability to take action that will support the NHS, regardless of their personal beliefs. During the pandemic, EveryDoctor began to invite all MPs to regular parliamentary briefings about various topics, bringing frontline doctors into contact with politicians to explain their concerns and to help lobby for changes that would protect staff and their patients too. During that period, a handful of Conservative politicians engaged with what we were doing, had telephone calls with us and signed up to our campaign pledge. But for the most part, when we sent MPs letters we would receive stock responses or slightly altered stock responses from Conservative politicians, or nothing at all. These stock responses are written by central communications teams, and they will often not directly answer the questions asked by us, or by constituents who are taking part in our campaign. They will more often than not be used as an opportunity for an MP to parrot whatever messaging the political party is hoping to disseminate about a topic at a given moment. This is frustrating at the best of times, but it was particularly galling to receive these responses during the middle of a pandemic, when every day counted and we were desperately hoping that politicians would step up and take action to help to make changes needed to safeguard the lives of NHS staff members and their vulnerable patients.

During the pandemic, we found it much easier to work with politicians from the other political parties, who seemed to have much more freedom to engage in our campaign in ways that were closely aligned with causes they felt strongly about, or issues that were strongly affecting their constituents and that they wanted to change. With the help of a large number of MPs from various political parties we were pivotal in securing some policy changes, including the provision of priority first-dose vaccines for frontline health and social care workers, and death-in-service benefits for the family members of frontline staff who had tragically died of COVID-19 after catching the virus in their workplaces.

The past couple of years in health campaigning have been frantic, with numerous situations arising that have required urgent public awareness raising, media work, and working with MPs. After a while, we got into a rhythm, and began to gain a sense of the core group of MPs for whom the NHS is a priority issue, and who would regularly engage with what we were doing, to help advocate for NHS staff and patients. There was the sense, for a time, that the Conservative Party's internal machinery was organising the responses of most of their MPs. They moved as a pack, and it was difficult to discern the personal ideologies of most. In contrast, the politicians of other parties appeared to have more scope to exercise their own political ideologies and judgement in calling for change. This situation (the lack of organised communication machinery, particularly within the Labour Party) benefited the NHS enormously. There were powerful calls from individual MPs or small groups who felt strongly about particular issues, and these resulted in important policy changes during the pandemic crisis.

But the landscape has shifted now. We began a campaign in autumn 2022 called #ReviveTheNHS, because we predicted that the NHS would be in a terrible state as we approached the winter months, and we put together five short-term policy changes that the government could implement in order to safeguard lives. At the time of writing we have run three parliamentary briefings, and over ten thousand people have sent letters to their MPs asking them to engage in the campaign. But we are finding now that we are receiving stock replies not just from Conservative politicians (which is what we had expected) but also from Labour MPs. A few of the latter are still engaged, mostly politicians who we know fairly well, who we have worked with in the past and for whom the NHS is a key issue that they feel very strongly about. But typically now, Labour MPs are sending stock responses to our emails that speak about Labour's long-term plans, should they win the next general election.

This is hugely problematic. We are running this campaign specifically to safeguard lives in the immediate term, and frankly are not interested in speaking about plans that won't come into being any time soon (if the next general election happens within the expected time-frame, it will be in late 2024 or early 2025). The current situation is an emergency. Every single day that passes sees more people dying unnecessarily within a public health-care system that isn't functioning. This isn't a situation that can wait a year or two; it needs action immediately.

The role of the political opposition is enormously important. It is extremely disappointing to see them focusing on their manifestos for the next election while this humanitarian crisis unfolds. Although it is the government that makes decisions concerning the NHS, setting budgets and so forth, the opposition has a key part to play too. The present administration has a great deal of autonomy due to it commanding such a large majority in the House of Commons. But the role of the opposition, as always, is to hold the government to account. The political landscape is ever-changing, and the landscape determines campaigners' ability to effect change. The state of a political party – how organised its messaging is, how much pressure the central organisa-tion is putting on individual MPs to toe the party line – can influence campaigners' ability to lobby for policy changes. And the current situation is affecting the NHS in a very negative way. Labour have organised themselves; they are pitching their manifesto for the next general election instead of reacting agilely and holding the current government to account about a situation that is costing many lives every day.

In the absence of robust, stringent accountability, Sunak and his government's actions are going largely unchallenged and unchecked. In November 2022, he appointed a private healthcare lobbyist called Bill Morgan[9] as a health policy advisor in Number 10 Downing Street. In December, he hosted a meeting with seven of the bosses of the UK's biggest private healthcare companies to discuss 'how to tackle the NHS backlog'.[10]

Beyond the influences of politicians' own political inclinations, and the priorities of the political party they represent, there are also external influences that may, or can, impact on politicians' decision-making. One would hope that the primary driver would be the opinions of the constituents that each politician serves as a Member of Parliament. These definitely do play a role. As part of our campaigning, we regularly build digital 'contact your MP' tools and help to mobilise large numbers of people who are concerned about particular issues to contact their MP. Some MPs do respond, particularly if sufficient numbers of constituents contact them at the same time. But there is increasing concern from many people that other interests may be being put before those of constituents or the general public.

Many people are worried about MPs holding second jobs. There are concerns about the amount of time and energy such jobs may take up, given that MPs are employed to represent their constituents (and a lot of the MPs I've engaged with have very full schedules to do so). MPs having second jobs has become somewhat normalised, because it's increasingly common, many now having at least one extra source of employment. But it's not just the existence of a second job that is cause for concern; it's the nature of that work.

Many were deeply disturbed when it was revealed that Matt Hancock had failed to declare a stake he owned in a private company that had won a contract to provide NHS services. Hancock was found to have broken the ministerial code on a technicality, when he failed to declare his 20 per cent ownership stake in a company called Topwood Ltd, which his brother and sister-in-law run.[11] Hancock engaged in a series of questionable decisions during his tenure as Health Secretary, including being featured within a paid-for advert about a private healthcare company called Babylon Health in the *Evening Standard*.[12] Opposition MPs raised concerns about whether Hancock had broken the ministerial code in doing so. And there were further questions when it was revealed that the backers of Babylon Healthcare later made a £10,000 donation to Hancock's Tory leadership campaign in 2019.[13] This was declared, and as such Hancock followed the rules and the donation was deemed to be acceptable.

We can't know for sure the power that any individual or employer holds over an individual's decision-making. And lots of these situations, involving second jobs for MPs, or taking on highly paid roles within the private healthcare sector, fall within the rules. The *Sunday Mirror* addressed the issue again in January 2023. In their piece, they stated that 'at least 28 Tory MPs and Lords have had ties to private health and medical groups, publicly accessible records reveal. There is no suggestion of wrongdoing.'[14] But there is a sense that the public is losing patience with the practice. It's one thing for something to be within the rules, and accepted as such by Parliament. It's another thing entirely for the public to accept it. The practice is being received particularly poorly at the moment because of the circumstances a lot of members of the public find themselves in; we are living through a cost-of-living crisis. Reports about MPs receiving huge sums of money to consult with private healthcare companies is leading to public criticism and disgust. Many people don't agree with politicians spending their time in this way; they feel it should be devoted to representing their constituents.

I speak to people online every day about the NHS, and the tone of communication has shifted recently. It feels as though a lot of people are growing increasingly frustrated at this behaviour from MPs, particularly where it relates to the private healthcare industry. The public is feeling the real effects of an inability to access the healthcare needed within the NHS. Many are anxious and scared. They are extremely concerned about the state of the NHS, and becoming increasingly aware of how entrenched privatisation now is within the service. Any suggestion of a link between politicians and the private healthcare industry is being received increasingly badly.

THE BETRAYAL

If we just look at the stark facts: there are 7.2 million people waiting on NHS waiting lists in England alone. There will be people struggling to cope with difficult symptoms, cancelled operations, worsening pain, in every single constituency in the UK. MPs should have enough on their plates serving those constituents, finding solutions to improve things, and lobbying for their interests.

Instead of becoming bogged down in endless discussions about the rules, the ministerial code, the details of whether or not a minister declared a stake in a private healthcare company or an NHS contract won by a family member, or any of this minutiae, it is time to stand back and evaluate this situation for what it is. There are three core NHS principles that should direct politicians' decision-making about its funding and strategic decisions concerning its future. They evidently have not been followed, because the NHS's management has veered off course so dramatically, so starkly, that hundreds of people are now needlessly dying every week as the service buckles.

And meanwhile, the media, the public, the politicians themselves are wasting valuable energy, time and attention discussing the issues outlined above, instead of focusing on patients. A combination of influences has led us to where we are today. A combination of self-interest, the promotion of the interests of others, allegiances to external sources – perhaps employers, friends or donors – and the pressure of one political party or another, vying for power. And meanwhile, the NHS is pushed into chaos. The car veers off course. The passengers are inside, and they are the ones harmed as politicians engage in this dereliction of their duties.

Even as all of this is going on, even as politicians make their questionable decisions and fail to take the action necessary to serve their constituents, NHS patients, some of those politicians still attempt to use the service as a vehicle to improve their personal brand. There's the sense from some of these politicians that by expressing their fondness for the service, they'll somehow be associated with the positive qualities that the NHS engenders in the eyes of the public. Matt Hancock provides a classic example of this. During his tenure as Health Secretary, he regularly pronounced his love for the NHS,[15] and wore an NHS badge with pride. His statements of support for the service rang hollow however, certainly among the medical community. Matt Hancock, after all, publicly promoted his own use of the private GP company Babylon, and said that he believed everyone in the UK should have access to their products. When Babylon began running NHS services, the company was widely and heavily criticised for cherry-picking healthy patients away from struggling NHS GP practices.[16]

The NHS is a vote-winner, and politicians use associations with the brand, and promises to improve it, to attract the support of the electorate. This is not a new situation, but it has become increasingly apparent as time has gone on and the service has deteriorated. In 2015, David Cameron said shortly after the election that 'the NHS will be in safe hands "for every generation to come"'.[17] Following the Brexit vote, there was speculation about whether Theresa May's government would deliver fully or partially on the pledge that had come from the 'vote Leave' campaign of delivering £350 million a week in NHS funding.[18] Jeremy Hunt, then Health Secretary, promised in 2015 that the number of GPs would increase by 5,000 by 2020.[19] Boris Johnson then made another pledge within his General Election manifesto in 2019: that he would increase the number of GPs by 6,000 by 2025.[20] Numbers of GPs have in fact fallen every single year since Jeremy Hunt made that pledge, and when Rishi Sunak took over as Prime Minister in autumn 2022 and set out his commitments, the pledge to increase GP numbers was notably absent.[21]

Perhaps the most prominent example of politicians' use of the NHS as a vote-winner was Boris Johnson's promise to build 40 new hospitals by 2030, made in the run-up to the General Election in 2019.[22] There was a lot of excitement about this promise. Many people believed this manifesto claim to mean that 40 entirely new hospitals would be built. It was a key plank during his election campaign, and hugely appealing to many voters.

Soon after Johnson became Prime Minister, the country was engulfed in the COVID-19 pandemic, and it was understandable that plans would be temporarily delayed. However, as we started to emerge from the most severe period of the pandemic, questions were asked about these hospitals, and concern built that they wouldn't be entirely new at all. Those concerns were well-founded. The BBC has recently reported that 'The National Audit Office says it "plans to start a value for money review of the New Hospitals Programme later this year" and report its findings in 2023.'[23] It has been revealed that in August 2021, the Department of Health and Social Care (DHSC) sent out a document to NHS Trusts describing what it referred to as 'key media lines' to use when discussing the new hospitals. These media lines describe a new hospital in three different ways: a whole new hospital (on existing NHS land or on a new site); a major refurbishment and alteration of all but the building frame or main structure of a hospital; or 'a major new clinical building on an existing site or a new wing of an existing hospital'.

Clearly, some of these building projects are not entirely new hospitals, as was claimed by Boris Johnson. The DHSC, however, instructed NHS Trusts via this document that there were a variety of schemes, but they 'must always be referred to as a new hospital'.[24] This sort of behaviour by the Department of Health and Social Care is extremely disappointing. There is a vast difference between a new clinical building on a hospital site, and an entirely new hospital. And the instruction to NHS Trusts to describe the situation in this way to the public feels very dishonest.

The BBC reported within the same article that they had emailed every NHS Trust involved, to find out which of these three categories their new building projects fit into. Some of the Trusts didn't reply to the BBC at all. Of the responses that the BBC did receive (34 in total), only five Trusts indicated that they were building a new hospital. Twelve explained that they would be building new hospital wings, and nine said that their project consisted of a rebuild of hospital buildings that already existed. The remaining respondents said they were unable to tell the BBC which category their new building would fit into.[25]

In February 2023, the *Observer* newspaper revealed that they had conducted their own investigation and discovered that only 10 of the 40 planned hospital projects have secured full planning permission. A boss at one of the NHS Trusts in question stated within the *Observer* piece: 'There's a 0% chance there's going to be 40 new hospitals by 2030.'[26]

We know, from the state of the service currently, that these promises have not been upheld, and it is difficult to view these instances as anything other than clever politicking. After all, large numbers of the public cast their vote during a general election based on the promises made in the party manifestos, and people care deeply about the NHS. If we can't trust what the politicians are saying, if their promises simply don't come to pass, where does that leave us? The situation feels particularly precarious right now, because things are in such peril. Promises from politicians going forward won't be able to use grandiose statements such as Cameron's, and any who, like Matt Hancock, attempted to wear an NHS badge in public today and claim their support for the service would probably face considerable ire. Things have spiralled into decline very quickly as these hollow promises have caused the public to place its faith in the wrong people.

The public doesn't take these manifesto promises lightly, and the medical community doesn't either. EveryDoctor was launched in early 2019, and so we were watching closely as the manifesto commitments were made public towards the end of the year. We painstakingly polled our members on their top priorities regarding the NHS, and created a scorecard, marking each political party against the promises they had or hadn't made, and we circulated this widely. It gained a degree of attention, so much so that one of the political parties got in touch, concerned that we hadn't adequately ascribed credit to their promises on one key area.

And EveryDoctor wasn't alone, isn't alone. A whole industry of political commentators and analysts exists, tasked with the scrutiny and assessment of what politicians are doing, and what they're planning. But if we can't trust the manifestos (and it feels increasingly that we cannot) then how can the public accurately decide who to vote for? One of my biggest concerns at the moment is that with one party (the Conservatives) making outlandish promises that they fail to fulfil, any other party carefully drawing up a manifesto that they will deliver on may fall short in the public's eyes, because their pronounced commitments might look less impressive. This situation isn't confined to healthcare of course; election season and manifesto promises are a minefield of bluffing and exaggeration, attacks and diversions from the full truth. But all this serves to demonstrate why the NHS should not be used as a political football. The exaggerations and the lies matter; the public is impacted on by all of this.

Alongside the manifesto promises, grand statements to secure votes to propel a politician into power, senior politicians in recent years have also made what feel like increasingly chaotic and inappropriate decisions regarding the NHS, the future of the service, and where the money should be spent. The most perplexing development, to my mind, is the rise of the 'NHS volunteer'. Personally, I don't agree there should be any volunteers within the NHS, because it is an essential public service and I worry about the sustainability and possible exploitation of such arrangements, where a person is working on behalf of the government but isn't being paid to do so. The phenomenon of NHS volunteers hasn't come out of nowhere. It has, however, expanded like never before in the last couple of years, through initiatives started by the current government.

During the COVID-19 pandemic, Matt Hancock was pivotal in bringing together what was referred to as a 'volunteer army', involving some 750,000 people who signed up within days to help vulnerable people.[27] Later on, when vaccines had become available, the *Sun* newspaper ran a campaign called 'Jabs Army', seeking 50,000 volunteers to help as stewards at vaccination centres.[28] One could argue that during an unprecedented national crisis, the involvement of volunteers was a positive thing, and undoubtedly they made a huge impact, even if some people found the messaging surrounding their recruitment jingoistic and inappropriate.

The situation hasn't stopped there, however. Sajid Javid (who was Health Secretary until the summer of 2022, two Health Secretaries ago), began asking people to sign up to a scheme as an 'NHS reservist' in March 2022.[29] The scheme essentially seems to provide basic training for a large pool of people, who are then employed on zero hours contracts to work in supporting roles at times of high pressure. The NHS in England is missing almost 10 per cent of its entire staff workforce currently.[30] Politicians should be focusing on employing permanent staff and supporting them properly to build sustainability within our health service, instead of creating a territorial army of NHS helpers in a bizarre echo of military service.

Along with the recruitment of volunteers during the height of the COVID-19 pandemic, a lot of attention was also drawn to 'NHS Charities Together', which is an independent charity that actually formed in 2000, but came to prominence during the pandemic when it launched 'the first ever national appeal for the NHS'. The organisation describes itself as 'working with a network of over 230 NHS Charities across the UK, to provide the extra support needed for staff, patients and communities'.[31] Not only is this organisation an oddity in its very existence, given that the NHS is a publicly funded service that should not require any associated charitable donations, but the organisation's website also claims that 'NHS Charities Together wants to build meaningful relationships with corporate partners'. The NHS was set up in the first place to do away with the reliance on philanthropy in the delivery of healthcare for our society. The existence of a charitable organisation propping up the service through corporate partnerships clashes with the very premise of our public healthcare system.

All of this is very powerful, however, in the framing of the NHS's role in the eyes of the public. It creates the sense that the NHS may not be able to cope at times of high pressure, and requires bolstering by an army of reserves, or donations. This plants the seed in people's minds that they cannot expect a comprehensive, all-encompassing health service all year round. The government is diminishing the expectations around what our public health service should provide.

When we consider the funding cuts, the hospital beds that have been lost, the staggering lack in capital investment that has left us with hospitals where in some places there is quite literally a hole in the roof, the spending on private consultancy firms to advise about the NHS in recent years is staggering. The amounts spent have varied enormously from year to year over the past decade, but as an example, in 2021 the government chose to spend almost £400 million on these private companies, in a bid to help make the NHS more 'efficient and cost-effective'.[32]

It is difficult to understand the logic of spending such vast sums of money on advice from these private businesses, when the government could be turning to the deep knowledge of local clinicians and national healthcare leaders who understand the needs of their patients and could provide excellent policy suggestions. A study in 2018 actually showed that the involvement of such management consultancies made the health service less efficient, not more.[33] Perhaps in a landscape of abundance, external advice might help. But when buildings are crumbling, surely it should be viewed as a luxury, to be possibly considered once we patch up the roofs and get the basic things right. Buildings that are robust. Enough staff. Staff who are paid appropriately, employed on proper contracts, work in good conditions, and do not require a charity dedicated to their support, or an army of volunteers to bolster the service.

Some of the policy suggestions from politicians in recent years have been nothing short of ludicrous; they will seemingly do nothing to support patients and staff, but instead helped to secure a bit of press coverage (presumably to serve some other end). During early 2021, amid a peak within the so-called 'culture wars', it seemed as if Union Jack flags were suddenly everywhere, promoted by Conservative politicians. To many people, this felt perplexing. But not to be left out, Matt Hancock was said to be an 'enthusiastic supporter' of flags flying at all NHS hospitals.[34] Bear in mind that, at the time, the horrors of the second major wave of COVID-19 were just abating. One might have expected that the Health Secretary had other priorities on his agenda.

For many years, it was difficult to explain the problems within the NHS to members of the general public, unless they had been taking an active interest in what had been going on. I remember an evening back in 2015, when our choir of junior doctors and others were doing some busking in central London and speaking to passers-by about what was happening to the NHS. When we got chatting to one man about underfunding and the threat of privatisation, he laughed at us and called us liars. He couldn't absorb the idea that the service was under threat, that it was being undermined. For many years throughout the 2010s, the service was struggling, but it held on because of the efforts of staff working incredibly hard, and because the Labour government until 2010 had invested so much money into the service that it provided a degree of resilience within the system for a while. Then the so-called winter crises began, each causing much consternation. But when these crises ebbed away, public awareness of what the politicians were doing diminished, and it was difficult to capture enough energy to hold them to account.

Now, however, things are different. It's interesting to witness a sea change in public opinion and awareness. I spend a lot of time speaking to thousands of people online about the NHS. The two issues of NHS privatisation and NHS underfunding, for example, used to be poles apart in people's minds. Many thought, in fact, that those discussing privatisation were conspiracy theorists, and politicians capitalised on this. As recently as 2022, when we were coordinating a campaign against the Health and Care Act 2022, several politicians attempted to discredit concerns that this Bill would lead to an acceleration in NHS privatisation.

And I think at the time, some people would have agreed with that. Those who weren't actively using the NHS weren't aware perhaps of the state of the service, or of the private outsourcing within it either. After all, private companies running NHS services put the NHS logo on the outside of their buildings. A lot of people don't even realise they're being treated by a private company. But now, things are changing fast. People are becoming increasingly aware of the actions of politicians; about the impact of their underfunding, their false promises, their false support, their discrediting of campaigners.

Politicians currently continue to press on with an agenda that is not serving patients' best interests. It became increasingly clear over the past 18 months that the situation was coming to a head. And yet still politicians seemed unwilling to tackle the situation head-on. In June 2022, Sajid Javid claimed that the NHS 'doesn't need any more money',[35] and Steve Barclay – briefly Health Secretary during the demise of Boris Johnson, before taking on the job again from Therese Coffey when Liz Truss crashed the UK economy – has similarly claimed that the NHS 'doesn't need cash'.[36]

Concerningly, the leader of the Labour Party, Keir Starmer, also seems to be promoting policies that do not tackle the current crisis, and that will not serve either the public or the continuation of the NHS in the long term. Starmer has a strong lead in opinion polls at present,[37] and many people believe that he will win the next election. He has been consistently vocal in his criticism of how the current government is handling the NHS, and was insistent during his campaign to become the elected leader of the Labour Party that he wanted to do things differently. Among the pledges he put forward to the membership of the Labour Party was that, if he were to be elected as Prime Minister, he would remove the private outsourcing of services within the NHS.[38] This was met with huge approval from many Labour Party members, and many of those NHS supporters who I speak to online every day voted for Starmer as leader specifically because of this pledge; it was enormously important to them.

It was extremely troubling for many, therefore, when Starmer recently said in an interview: 'there is some private provision within the NHS and we're likely to have to continue with that'.[39] Some have suggested that Starmer believes that breaking his election promise could help him to win a general election. His shadow health secretary, Wes Streeting, has also recently explained that he sees a role for the private sector as 'one of the levers' for tackling the long NHS waiting lists.[40]

Many members of the public are becoming unhappy with politicians' behaviour, and there have been several prominent examples of members of the public holding them to account when they visit NHS facilities. In October 2022, a hospital patient challenged Rishi Sunak over nurses' pay.[41] In December 2022, during a hospital visit, Health Secretary Steve Barclay was confronted by the mother of a sick girl who told him that 'NHS staff are "worked to the bone", and the government is doing "terrible damage" to families on waiting lists'.[42]

Because of the power that is placed in the hands of politicians (particularly at times like this, when the ruling party commands a large majority), politicians hold great power over the direction of the NHS. This has enabled them to use the service as a vote-winner, a badge of honour, even as they take steps to damage the service. Their failure to stick to the NHS constitution and take decisions in the best interests of patients is clear. But things are changing, and it feels like there's going to be a wide-scale reckoning of their actions.

3

THE METHOD

Assessing what's gone wrong with the NHS goes beyond individuals. It's not just a question of who's to blame, but also what's to blame. We don't appear to have functional mechanisms within our society to hold politicians to account as they take successive steps to break down our public healthcare system. The current problems within the NHS fall into two main categories: problems with the service's structure and function because of the reforms over the past 40 years, and those due to government budget cuts, which are undermining the safe delivery of healthcare. It is useful to separate the issues associated with the service's demise into these two broad categories, because it helps to explain why the collapse of the NHS started slowly and is now accelerating at breakneck speed.

The NHS's structure and the way it functions have changed remarkably over the past 40 years. Successive governments implemented NHS reforms that have diminished the responsibility politicians hold towards patients, and have increasingly handed that responsibility over to local NHS services. They have also gradually opened the NHS up to external providers, including private companies. These include companies that specialise in dermatology, or surgery, or even eye tests through the high-street opticians Specsavers.[1] These providers can bid for and win NHS contracts to run public services, and take taxpayers' money to do so. All of this has resulted in our public healthcare system becoming progressively fragmented, with a churn of external providers running short-term contracts, which results in differing patient experiences across the country, and also different experiences over time.

Particularly for patients with chronic conditions, this matters. They may get to know one team delivering their healthcare, only to find that the local service has changed hands and they'll now be managed by different staff. On paper, they're receiving the same care. In reality, they're not. Relationships within healthcare matter. Degradation of staff–patient relationships has an impact. This issue doesn't receive enough attention, but in this way the proliferation of short-term contracts goes beyond the contracts, partnerships and business deals. There have also been various administrative problems. Some patients have explained that they have accidentally dropped down waiting lists or off a list altogether in the chaos and bureaucracy of one healthcare team transferring responsibility to the next.

EveryDoctor decided to build an interactive map showing the extent of NHS outsourcing across the UK,[2] and we've found that there are thousands of these external providers, mostly in England. The example that has stuck out for me the most is Specsavers. They're not alone in being a chain; lots of the companies and organisations involved hold multiple NHS contracts delivering patient services. But there's something about the company's existence as a high-street shop that stands out. They're a household name, a business with recognisable branding and adverts, and their premises aren't simply used for the delivery of healthcare. They sell glasses and other accessories. Presumably, if a person went to Specsavers for an NHS-funded eye test, they would be served by Specsavers employees, and walk through a showroom full of things for sale. It seems like a strange place to be receiving public funds and running a public service.

The reforms that are changing the structure of the NHS continue to evolve, the most recent one only coming into place in July 2022, with the Health and Care Act 2022.[3] Described by the then Health Secretary Sajid Javid as 'the most significant change to the healthcare system in a decade',[4] we have yet to see the full impact of its changes. But essentially this new Act follows the trajectory of the reforms that have come before. It has further fragmented services in England, this time into 42 'Integrated Care Systems', led by Integrated Care Boards.[5] The government quietly brought these major changes into being at a time when many people were distracted by other concerns, such as energy prices and the cost-of-living crisis.

During the Bill's journey through Parliament, politicians repeatedly spoke of their desire to reduce the 'bureaucracy'[6] involved in awarding NHS contracts – words that raised alarm bells for many people. Checks and balances in awarding NHS contracts are absolutely necessary. When such a contract is given to a provider, a huge amount of taxpayer money is entrusted to them. And what's more, NHS staff have raised concerns that the new Integrated Care Boards do not have sufficient representation of local clinical staff who understand the needs of their respective patient populations. Campaigners are very worried that NHS contracts could be awarded with less due diligence from now on, and that those deciding on who to award them to will have insufficient expertise to make good decisions on behalf of patients.

These structural changes, fragmenting the service and breaking down relationships, have been going on in the background for several decades now. But while they were felt in many small ways previously, it has been the 'austerity cuts' since 2010 that have truly exposed the problems with these NHS reforms. Cuts were made across public services from 2010, in the fall-out following the 2007/08 financial crisis. Since the austerity years began, the NHS has felt like a public healthcare system in steady decline.[7]

There have been various announcements of increased investment in the NHS, which have been accompanied with great media fanfare on each occasion, but these investments have never matched the funding required in real terms. I had one particularly frustrating conversation in 2019 with a leading journalist at a national newspaper who couldn't understand why EveryDoctor was campaigning for additional funding. He was extremely well informed about UK politics, and was under the impression that the government had made significant efforts to re-invest in the health service. The NHS becomes more and more expensive to run every year for a variety of reasons. As described by the BBC, 'Average annual UK health spending in real terms rose by more than 4% in the 1960s, 70s and 90s. It went up to 6% in the 2000s.'[8] During the 2010s, the Conservative government cut this to 1.6 per cent.[9] We're now in a terrible state, and as the NHS Confederation explained in July 2022, the NHS in England faced a funding hole of between £4 billion and £9.4 billion in real terms in 2022 alone.[10]

Some of the structural problems with the NHS reforms were masked for a long time because of injections of funding, which kept the service running well despite the increasing fragmentation of its structure. When the funding was stripped away from 2010 onwards, it revealed some of the worst elements of these reforms. And as budgets were slashed and local healthcare services were forced to cut essential parts of their services, they then took the blame for many of the inevitable failures that ensued. Many of the hospitals that have struggled the most are ones that took on PFI projects, often 20 years earlier.

Private finance initiatives (PFI) were schemes whereby the government could borrow money from the private sector in order to pay for the design, build and maintenance of various types of new infrastructure, including roads and hospitals. The money was then paid back with interest over many years to those who financed the work. It was a scheme that frankly was too good to be true, and politicians were warned about this at the time of the inception of the PFI schemes, which mostly began during Blair's tenure as Prime Minister. Many could foresee the incredible interest payments that would fall to NHS Trusts, and were worried about the impact this would have on NHS services and their patients.[11]

This, of course, came to pass. Government figures released in 2018 show that the PFI schemes involving the NHS had a value of £12.8 billion, but by the time the debt is finally cleared (sometime around 2050) the taxpayer will have paid out £80 billion for these hospitals and other facilities. The cost has been astronomical, and has not fallen equally across the country. A report by the Institute for Public Policy Research (IPPR) think-tank has shown that the PFI contract taken on by Barts Health Trust in London, which involved an initial outlay of almost £1.2bn, is the largest by value in the NHS in England. This enormous sum paid for the new Royal London hospital in Mile End,[12] which opened in 2012 and has 845 beds. The cost to the Trust has been extraordinary. Barts Health spends £116m every single year in paying off the debt it has incurred, and this figure represents 7.66 per cent of its total annual income.

As the *New Statesman* reported in May 2022, some NHS Trusts are paying more on PFI repayments than they are on their total annual medicines bill.[13] An analysis of NHS finances during the year 2019/20 shows, for example, that Sherwood Forest Hospitals NHS Foundation Trust spent more than double on PFI repayments than it did on drugs. The situation is horrifying. And that's not all. The PFI schemes often involved clauses that stated that the hospitals had to continue to pay particular private providers for maintenance of the infrastructure. For NHS hospitals, this involved such things as fixing door handles, resetting alarms and installing air fresheners. Such things are part of the day-to-day functioning of hospitals. These agreements, which forced the hospitals to pay the private companies for maintenance, meant that the private companies could create a monopoly system and charge huge sums of money for very basic maintenance and repairs. The *Daily Mail* ran an exposé on the situation, which highlighted some unbelievable examples of exploitation of these contracts. In one example, an NHS Trust was charged £242 to change the padlock on a garden gate. In another, perhaps the most extraordinary example found, a Trust was charged £13,704 to install three lights in a garden.[14]

The government finally acknowledged the damaging nature of the PFI schemes, and stopped new projects being entered into in 2018.[15] But despite multiple appeals to the government to pay off the PFI debt now, in order to wipe the slate clean and reduce the interest repayments that will continue to burden the NHS for decades, it has resisted this. The NHS Trusts affected have become the worst victims of the NHS reforms. Saddled with enormous debt repayments year after year, they have also had to absorb austerity cuts like everywhere else. There has been barely any attempt from the Conservative government to step in and assist these services. The result has been inescapable spirals of failure for some NHS Trusts. Struggling services fail on performance metrics, become increasingly stressful to work in, and face staff shortages as employees leave to work elsewhere.

Through our work with EveryDoctor, we receive testimony from NHS workplaces all over the country, telling us what is happening, alerting us to problems. And the same hospital names come up time and time again. I've come to know which I'm most likely to be messaged about; typically Trusts with long-standing financial problems. The staff working within these hospitals are just as well trained, and work just as hard as anywhere else in the country. But I hear time and time again about doctors in these hospitals being pushed into working huge numbers of extra hours, often with inadequate payment. I'm told about staff arriving at hospital for a day shift, only to learn that there'll be no one to cover the night shift, so they're forced to go home, sleep for a few hours and then return. I'm sent emails that consultants have received from management, putting them under enormous pressure to discharge patients. It's a hopeless situation, and the government repeatedly fails to step in and help these hospitals, pay off the debt and put them into a more financially robust position, thus supporting patients and staff. The NHS should be providing an equal service everywhere, but these situations change the landscape considerably, and have placed some local populations at a significant disadvantage within our public healthcare system.

Meanwhile, external providers who are running NHS services are able to simply end their contracts when things go wrong. A private healthcare company called Circle did just that. Circle was the first private company to run an NHS hospital, Hinchingbrooke Hospital in Cambridgeshire.[16] The company had won the contract to run the hospital under the leadership of Ali Parsa. As the *Financial Times* reported in 2015, the Chief Inspector for hospitals, Sir Mike Richards, was hours away from publishing a damning report into the state of the hospital when Circle pulled out of their contract. The inspectors had found 'serious concerns, surrounding staffing and risks to patient safety particularly in the A&E department and medical care'.[17] The company was just three years into its ten-year NHS contract when it pulled out. Circle specifically cited the 10 per cent cut in funding to their hospital as a reason they had decided to end the contract, along with an increase in the numbers of A&E patients attending the hospital. The upheaval to the service involved in this situation cannot be underestimated, and there are broader implications too. If private companies can swoop in, take on lucrative contracts paid by taxpayer money, and then exit when things go wrong, where is the accountability towards patients?

Interestingly (and disturbingly), Ali Parsa was later involved in another high-profile failed project with the NHS. He is the Chief Executive of Babylon, the private healthcare company that disgraced former Health Secretary Matt Hancock publicly endorsed on a number of occasions.[18] Babylon embarked on several projects within the NHS, including a digital healthcare app for primary care called GP at hand.[19] This project has been widely criticised by campaigners. The service allows patients to de-register from their NHS practice and join GP at hand instead, where they can access online appointments with Babylon GPs. As indicated earlier, Babylon has been accused of cherry-picking certain groups of NHS patients away from NHS GP surgeries – those who tend to have fewer and less complex healthcare needs – while leaving clinically complex patients to be managed in the NHS. Babylon Healthcare also embarked on three contracts with NHS Trusts. As *Wired* reported in August 2022, 'Babylon Health cancelled its last hospital contract with the UK National Health Service (NHS) eight years early, with CEO Ali Parsa calling such projects "a distraction" that aren't lucrative enough to bother with as the company seeks to cut costs.'[20]

These examples reveal how fragile the relationships between private companies and the NHS can be. They are business relationships, and as soon as conditions become unfavourable, either because of increased pressures or due to reduced funding, the private healthcare company is able to extricate itself from its obligations. This goes against the very premise of the NHS. We have a public healthcare system to provide comprehensive care to all. Not only did Ali Parsa fail to deliver on his responsibilities with Circle Healthcare, he was also allowed to embark on further NHS contracts that have subsequently been abandoned when they didn't prove sufficiently profitable. To think that he was publicly endorsed on multiple occasions by the Health Secretary of the time is terrible; it should have been a national scandal.

And yet it wasn't. The situation received minimal attention in the UK press. And where is Matt Hancock now? He is serving as an Independent MP, having been disgraced out of his position as Health Secretary for breaking COVID rules, and then later deciding to abandon his constituents to take part in reality TV show *I'm a Celebrity ... Get Me Out of Here!*[21] Hancock has decided not to stand at the next UK general election, and in the letter he wrote to Rishi Sunak about his future intentions, he said, 'I have discovered a whole new world of possibilities which I am excited to explore.' One hopes tentatively that none of these possibilities involve managing a public service.

Over the last couple of years, the pandemic has thrown up many lucrative ways for private healthcare companies to benefit financially from the public purse. As one example, in the spring of 2020, the UK government decided to 'block purchase' private hospital capacity, to enable it both to borrow the staff and equipment of these hospitals and to use the facilities themselves if the NHS became completely overwhelmed. At the end of 2020, the *Health Service Journal* revealed that two-thirds of this private hospital capacity, which is thought to have cost the taxpayer £400 million a month, was left unused for months on end over the summer.[22] This represents an incredible waste of money, which could have been used to fund NHS services at a time when the service was coming under increasing pressure.

The *Mirror* reported in January 2021 that, regardless of this waste, yet more private hospitals would be paid 'millions of pounds' to take NHS patients for the next three months, due to pressures on the service.[23] Another similar deal was struck with the private sector in January 2022, earning private healthcare companies between £75 million and £90 million a month in early 2022,[24] according to the *Guardian*. And as well as these vast sums of money being spent, with little attention being given to the efficiency of this spending, there have even been questions raised about the proportion of the total NHS budget that the Department of Health and Social Care funnels into the private sector each year. The mainstream media, along with the prominent independent think-tank The King's Fund, seem to have accepted the figures offered by the Department of Social Care, which state that in recent years, around 7 per cent of the total budget has gone to the independent sector.[25] This 7 per cent figure is in fact regularly used by people on social media as 'evidence' to 'prove' to campaigners that we are overreacting when we speak about our concerns regarding the escalation of NHS privatisation.

But a blog post by David Rowland (Director of the independent think-tank the Centre for Health and the Public Interest), published in 2019 by the LSE,[26] points out the enormous flaws in this presentation of the data. Within its published figures, the Department of Health and Social Care has excluded various important items from its calculations. Rowland estimates that in the financial year 2018/19, if spending on NHS GPs was excluded, NHS England spent 18 per cent, not 7 per cent, of its total budget on the independent sector. Rowland also demonstrated within his piece that the figures have risen significantly between the years 2013/14 and 2018/19, an increase that has been primarily driven by a corresponding increase in the purchase of care by the NHS from non-NHS providers.

Every government has a large degree of power over what happens in the NHS, but some have more power than others. And this comes down to their parliamentary majority. The current Conservative government won a huge majority of 80 seats in the 2019 General Election that saw Boris Johnson become Prime Minister, the biggest Tory majority since 1987.[27] Those governments that command a large majority of MPs in the House of Commons have a significant advantage in proceeding with legislative changes. This has benefited the current government enormously in pushing many Bills through Parliament, including the Health and Care Act 2022. It has been a very difficult time for campaigners on all sorts of causes, and this situation looks set to continue for the rest of this government's tenure.

However, in a functioning democracy, there are various societal mechanisms that temper the power of any government to create new legislation. It doesn't all come down to votes within Parliament, because if the views of the public are set firmly against the actions of a government, it is sometimes put under sufficient pressure to withdraw plans or make policy U-turns. And there are other mechanisms for holding the government to account – mechanisms that are enormously important in scrutinising the government's actions, providing analysis, building public awareness and enabling stakeholders and experts to exert influence on the direction of travel.

Returning, first, to the views of the general public, if the government is attempting to push through a change that is not in the public's interest, and the public is well aware of the context and detail of the situation, it is relatively easy to draw energy together and formulate collective action against what the government is proposing.

Some of this context will be the public's own experiences (for example, at the moment, the public doesn't need to be educated about the realities of the cost-of-living crisis, already living through the experience and understanding what's going on), and some will have been absorbed from other sources, most notably the media.

The media, broadly, has failed to hold the government to account for what it has done to the NHS. Most news organisations are, themselves, politically positioned, with a solid stance on their views concerning public services, which influences their reporting. Unless it's a national emergency, where normal practice is suspended and the evolving situation tends to be covered more impartially, they'll select stories to report on that support the view they want to promote to their readership. In this way, some UK media outlets can be relied upon to print story after story about how the service is wasteful and takes up too much taxpayer money, while others inform us of the lack of funding this government has assigned to the NHS, or the real-terms pay cuts that staff have endured for years. On any given day, if you google 'NHS news' you will be met with a patchwork of conflicting information that can be very difficult to navigate. News stories blaming staff for problems bump up against articles describing how the government is to blame for the things that are deteriorating within the health service.

What the media is not doing very successfully is providing analytical coverage of the development of NHS problems over time. These problems are long-standing, and we find ourselves in our current situation because of layered decisions one on top of another, going back decades. It's not enough to announce a new pot of funding for the NHS, or write an isolated article about some bed cuts. It doesn't successfully explain to people what is going on, the big picture.

And to make matters worse, many of us consume our media in small snapshots now; short pieces constructed around a soundbite or a single graph shared online. A number of the national news outlets operate behind a paywall, so lots of people don't even click to read an article before sharing. We simply validate our existing views by reading a headline, and by spreading the information further across the internet via a 'like' or a 'retweet'. There's not a lot of time for reflection, either by the journalists or by their audiences. We're given just enough information to become intrigued or inflamed, and then it's on to the next thing. Snapshot after snapshot within a rapidly spinning news cycle. Many journalists operating within this frenetic arena are simply chasing the next bite-size chunk of rage that can be parcelled up and shipped out, in the hope that it will go viral.

The articles and broadcasts are often reductive in nature, overly simplifying the information to make it digestible. And they focus on the here and now, ignoring the intentional stepwise decisions that have brought us here. The current coverage of NHS waiting lists exemplifies this style of reporting. Predictable as clockwork, on the day that the latest NHS stats are announced, the national news outlets pepper social media with yellow 'breaking news' banners. The articles detail the number of people waiting for hospital treatment across the UK, the average ambulance waiting times, the number of patients waiting for longer than 12 hours in A&E for a hospital admission.

As we emerged from the pandemic, and waiting lists, together with waiting times for ambulances and in A&E, got longer and longer, the media had an opportunity to provide some analysis of what was happening. It was necessary; the public was struggling to gain a sense of the detail and nuance of the situation. Instead, every single month as the NHS stats have been announced, the media spotlight has been temporarily trained on the ambulance bays of A&E car parks, for some perfunctory reporting on the situation. Some of the national news outlets might even set up a rolling newsfeed on their website. We'll be shown a few pictures of the inside of A&E waiting rooms, and staff are interviewed, but it's generally surface-level reporting, acknowledging the burnout and the crowding and the dissatisfaction of patients, but not really digging into why these things have happened, not properly. Blame is often attributed to the pandemic, which is certainly one of the causes of these problems, but it's not the only one. We're not told about the lack of capital investment in the buildings that has contributed to the crowding. We're not told about the piecemeal fragmentation of the service through successive reforms, infiltrating the service with privatisation, and we're not even usually reminded of the chronic underinvestment in the service that has stripped it of so much that it used to provide.

THE METHOD

The media pieces, which are churned out month after month, provide some comparison of the numbers themselves, but it's mostly meaningless, comparing this month with last month, or three months earlier. There's very little broad analysis of the numbers over the last ten years, to successfully examine the true scale of politicians' decisions, their small, intentional, relentless decisions to dismantle our public healthcare system.

And then, as quickly as the yellow-bannered alerts arrive on our social media newsfeeds, they're gone again. We can expect sporadic reporting on tragic situations where patients die in the backs of ambulances, or particularly harrowing cases of ambulances not turning up to dying patients' houses, but none of it touches the edges of this crisis. None of it captures the grinding reality of what it means to be denied the healthcare that patients pay for through their taxes, none of it captures the new barriers that are being thrown up against people accessing the care they need.

The need for sensationalism and click-bait worsens this landscape further. When I spoke to one high-profile journalist about this recently, they explained to me that their news desk would only allow journalists to write stories about the NHS if the detail within the piece was sufficiently 'worse' than in previous coverage. And this presents a problem. NHS crises don't come out of nowhere; the situation has developed because of a series of failures in many different areas that were predicted and predictable. It isn't made up of new, short-term emergencies that can create compelling content. It grinds on and has been doing so for years, getting incrementally worse, to the detriment of everyone who relies upon the service. What we need is proper analysis and nuanced, thoughtful reporting that scrutinises the government and holds it to account for its actions.

This patchy coverage of the political trajectory that is causing the demise of our public healthcare system is a huge problem. The media is one of the key mechanisms within our society that could wield influence over the actions of successive governments regarding the NHS. Major UK media outlets are enormously powerful. During the COVID-19 pandemic, we saw the government embark on U-turns time and time again when they were held to account by newspapers and campaigners, and realised they were falling out of favour with the public. The most high-profile examples, such as the two separate U-turns on the provision of free school meals[28] and the U-turns on school closures during the height of the pandemic, had an impact on millions of UK citizens.

The media itself, of course, has its own inherent conflicts and compromises. The vast majority of our national print newspapers are owned by just four families, who hold enormous political influence. And as reported, 'from the point at which Boris Johnson became Prime Minister in July 2019 to the end of September 2020, three billionaire press owners (Murdock, Rothermere and Barclay), and their representatives, had more meetings [with him] than all the rest of the UK media combined'.[29] It is perhaps unlikely, therefore, that scrutiny of NHS privatisation will be increasing any time soon.

THE METHOD

And the media isn't alone in its failure to raise awareness among the public and hold successive governments to account. There should also be mechanisms whereby experts, and organisations representing particular groups of people and causes, have a say in the public discourse around topics of national importance. This is important; it helps everyone to understand things better, for good decisions to be made.

We have medical organisations and charities that should fulfil this role, and provide scrutiny and accountability in relation to the government's behaviour. Some organisations do perform this role extremely effectively; for example, the Royal College of Emergency Medicine's report on A&E crowding in November 2021, called 'Crowding and its Consequences', was incredibly powerful.[30] The *Guardian* newspaper covered the report, which stated that 'an estimated 4,519 people in England died in 2020–21 as a direct result of people receiving less than ideal care while delayed in A&E waiting to start treatment in the hospital'.[31] As the vice-president of the college, Dr Adrian Boyle, explained in the piece, 'to say this figure is shocking is an understatement. Quite simply, crowding kills.' This report secured widespread coverage and was a hugely important piece of work, highlighting the direct consequences to patients of the pressures within the NHS.

The Royal College of Emergency Medicine is not alone in highlighting the problems with the NHS. Many organisations are working extremely hard to draw attention to them, sometimes publicly and sometimes behind the scenes, through government committees and the submission of reports into various areas of concern. The NHS Confederation,[32] in particular at the moment, is providing crucial analysis on a range of issues including NHS funding shortfalls and the impact of the energy crisis. But it's not enough, and it's an uphill struggle for many of these individuals and groups to gain the widespread coverage and influence that their information deserves.

Some organisations also face limitations on the degree to which they can openly criticise the UK government. For example, despite being enormously powerful within the UK medical profession, and being held in high regard because of their depth of knowledge and expertise on so many topics, the medical Royal Colleges are charities. Charities are severely restricted by law in their ability to campaign in the 12 months leading up to a general election, for fear of them wielding political influence.

This is hugely problematic, and some charities have referred to it as a 'gagging law', calling for it to be removed by the next UK government.[33] There have been instances recently where charities, including the RNLI[34] and the National Trust,[35] have been targeted by politicians and newspaper columnists and others for ostensibly becoming 'too political'. Some fear that many charities could lose their charitable status, and as a result some charities stay silent when they'd like to speak up.

This system of expertise, of organisations offering their experience and guidance to politicians for the betterment of our society, relies on politicians engaging in the discourse. There is a sense at the moment that this willingness to listen has been lost. Michael Gove famously said during the Brexit campaign that people had 'had enough of experts'. It seems more likely that this is true of the government rather than the public.

EveryDoctor ran a large national campaign as the Health and Care Bill 2021 proceeded through Parliament,[36] and as part of this campaign we and others sent a great deal of correspondence to MPs of all political parties to establish their thoughts and intended actions. We opposed the Bill because we were (and are) concerned that the ensuing Act would lead to an acceleration in NHS privatisation.

It is very difficult to frame a campaign about a presumed outcome that will happen sometime in the future. You're speaking about something that hasn't yet come to pass, and this is leveraged against you by opposing political forces. So it was a difficult campaign to run. And it was especially difficult for the reasons listed above; despite privatisation having heavily infiltrated the NHS in a number of ways, many UK media outlets don't discuss it, analyse it or scrutinise the situation. And so we have relied on the public, building up a huge online community of people who are concerned and want to discuss NHS privatisation and campaign against it.

It was extremely interesting to watch how things unfolded during our campaign against the Health and Care Act 2022. Before the Bill returned to the House of Commons for its second reading, we coordinated over twelve thousand people writing to MPs within a couple of days. We then asked those people to send any replies they received back to us. We wanted to see how each political party was framing the issues, and whether we would receive stock responses from politicians 'toeing the party line' or whether individual MPs would construct their own responses to constituents. It can be useful to assess a range of responses, because this enables campaign organisations to identify 'targets'; MPs who will be amenable to engage and work together on particular points of legislation.

Many MPs simply ignored the emails they were sent by their constituents. And perhaps worse, constituents of a lot of Conservative MPs were sent endless platitudes and reassurances. Many of these responses derived from a stock reply that we presumed was drafted within a central press department. Sometimes the Conservative responses went beyond mere platitudes and took a different tack, seemingly attempting to discredit our campaign. We were sent numerous emails from constituents, saying that 'it is irresponsible scaremongering to suggest that Integrated Care Systems are being used to support privatisation'.[37] There have been moments during our campaigning when these insinuations of inaccuracy or accusations of our own 'politicking' have caused me to question our own logic and rationale; it is disconcerting to be questioned in this way. We are fastidious about our fact-checking, and when we receive criticisms of this nature, we fastidiously check again, ensuring we haven't overstated facts or shared an inaccuracy. But the facts, here, are very clear. The World Health Organization's 1995 definition of privatisation within healthcare is 'a ... process in which non-government actors become increasingly involved in the financing and/or provision of health care services'.[38] And this is exactly what is happening in the NHS.

The most obvious group to question the government's actions around NHS privatisation would be the political opposition in the House of Commons, which currently is the UK Labour Party, led by Keir Starmer, and so our hopes rode on the responses from Labour Party MPs. But while there is a faction within the party that is ardently against NHS privatisation and speaks up frequently about its dangers and pitfalls, this group of MPs is not currently the dominant force within the Labour Party. When we were running our campaign against the Health and Care Act 2022, I was actually surprised at the low number of Labour politicians who chose to become actively involved. During Jeremy Corbyn's leadership, the renationalisation of the NHS and the removal of NHS privatisation was a key item on Labour's agenda.[39] It appears to have slipped down the priority list now that Keir Starmer is in charge.[40]

The level of focus that UK politicians across the political spectrum are placing upon NHS privatisation, or the lack thereof, was put into starkest relief for me when we attempted to bring politicians together to help them set up an All Party Parliamentary Group against NHS privatisation. I was hopeful, at the time, that even within the Conservative Party we would be able to find some politicians who did not agree with the current direction of travel and would be willing to engage in cross-party working on this topic. Sadly I was wrong. Despite enormous effort, we could not find a single current Conservative

MP who wanted to help lead the APPG, and when we attempted to find a Conservative peer, things were just as challenging. In order to set up an APPG, you must have a member of the ruling political party as part of the leadership. I had various phone calls with peers who kindly lent me some of their valuable time.

I eventually thought that I had found one Conservative peer who would help; he was extremely thoughtful and helpful, and could see the merit in setting up this working group. However, he was also very elderly, and he eventually decided not to become involved, because he no longer travelled regularly to Westminster and wasn't sure how much longer he would remain active within the House of Lords. I felt quite despondent about this; about the structure of our political system. This gentleman was enormously helpful and I cannot fault his willingness to engage in and thoughtfully discuss the situation. But surely something is wrong with our political system if a member of our second chamber chooses not to engage in a campaign because they are unable to attend the chamber regularly? Those with positions of power should be utilising them, hopefully for the public good.

It was sobering to realise that within an entire political party, which commanded an enormous majority in the House of Commons, there was not a single MP or peer who wanted to set up and help lead a group opposing the privatisation of the NHS.

Politicians of the past 40 years have benefited from the various limitations and compromises within the structures that exist to hold them accountable, and things are particularly bad right now, with a quiet political opposition, a complicit media that doesn't effectively hold them to account, and the effective silencing of experts who are being ignored when they warn about the implications of decisions on patients, on staff and on the integrity of the service. It's a difficult landscape to campaign within at the moment, with organisations that are stymied in their pushback by laws, by bullying, by unfair attacks in the media or even by the apparent coordinated infiltration onto their boards of those with extremist agendas.

And things are likely to get even more challenging. At the same time that the government pushed through the Health and Care Act 2022, it also pushed the Police, Crime, Sentencing and Courts Bill through Parliament. This Bill will make it much harder for groups of people to congregate and protest in the UK. In the BBC's reporting on the Bill, it noted that 'Parliament's Joint Committee on Human Rights said the proposals are "oppressive and wrong"'.[41] The committee accused the government of trying to create 'new powers in areas where the police already have access to powers and offences which are perfectly adequate'.

All of these developments are incredibly concerning for all UK citizens. It's certainly so for campaigners. We use various tactics to raise public awareness about key pieces of information; for example, we attempt to hold politicians to account for their links to NHS privatisation, or call attention to politicians' failings to keep workers safe in their working environments, by engaging in public actions. These actions often involve us working closely with artists, with photographers, with animators, videographers and graphic designers to create imagery that is powerful and compelling, and in our work (just as with so many other campaign organisations, now and in the past) we try to draw as much attention as possible to what we're doing. In the course of EveryDoctor's work and in the campaigns I've been a part of previously, we've filmed a music video opposite Westminster, we've projected imagery onto hospitals and buildings of key institutions, we've even projected imagery onto Parliament itself. We've hired ad vans and have photographed them driving around Westminster, or have parked them outside the headquarters of private healthcare companies. During the pandemic we created masks with our social media hashtags on, and we've made campaign stickers and posters, t-shirts, and many other things. Items to help us make as much impact and noise as we can, to raise awareness and start conversations.

This is important. And this is under threat. There is huge concern among campaigners and the wider public at the moment that the ability of activists and others to speak up, protest, congregate and express their dissatisfaction with the trajectory of political travel is under threat due to the Police, Crime, Sentencing and Courts Act 2022. And beyond this, another Bill is causing huge concern as well. The National Security Bill. As the *Guardian* put it in an article written in January 2023: 'An offence is deemed to have occurred if a person "engages in conduct that it is reasonably possible may materially assist a foreign intelligence service" and "knows, or ought reasonably to know, that it is reasonably possible their conduct may materially assist" such a spy agency.' Many have considerable reservations about the far-reaching impact of the Bill. As explained by Guy Black, the deputy chair of Telegraph newspapers: 'The UK's proposed national security bill could have a "chilling effect" on investigative journalism because it sets too low a bar on what constitutes spying.' One of the major worries is that the Bill could 'potentially criminalise' investigative reporters and whistle-blowers who are bringing important information into the public domain.[42] This may have an impact across all sectors, including healthcare. It is already difficult for healthcare workers to speak up at work; there are barriers to doing so that many staff struggle with. A Bill that could implicate people speaking up could hamper the public understanding of what is happening in the NHS. We are watching developments with concern.

It is important that people understand what is happening; more important now than at any time in the NHS's long history. Politicians have found it too easy to make empty promises. Margaret Thatcher claimed that 'the NHS is safe in our hands'[43] before creating an internal marketplace within the service. Tony Blair's election manifesto in 1997 claimed that only Labour could 'save the NHS',[44] and he then proceeded to enable many of the PFI projects that burden the NHS with billions of pounds of debt repayment every single year. And David Cameron, not to be outdone, declared in his first speech following the General Election in 2015 that the NHS 'will be safe in his hands "for every generation to come"'.[45] And while politicians have evaded proper scrutiny, dismissing concerns and making empty statements, their real work happens behind the scenes.

Tucked away from the noise, quietly ensconced in boardrooms, the UK government is getting on with that work, planning its next steps in the dismantlement of the NHS as a publicly funded, publicly run healthcare system, and its reinvention as a corporate machine, funnelling increasing amounts of money into the private sector. Boris Johnson recruited Samantha Jones into a senior post in Downing Street in April 2021. She was initially recruited as the Prime Minister's most senior advisor on NHS transformation and social care. Jones wasn't new to this; she had originally worked as an NHS nurse and had moved into NHS management, working as a Chief Executive in two separate NHS hospital Trusts. But it is her sidestep into the private healthcare industry that causes concern. Jones had become the CEO of Centene, the UK arm of the US healthcare giant Operose. Centene, as described by the *Guardian*, 'recently became one of the largest primary care providers in England, with 58 practices and more than 500,000 patients'.[46]

Samantha Jones was promoted in February 2022 to become Number 10's first ever Chief Operating Officer. It remains to be seen what impact she will have, but even her new job title brings the impression of a business agenda. Her recruitment is certainly not the first time that an individual with experience within the healthcare insurance industry has made their way close to the corridors of UK power. Simon Stevens, who ran NHS England between 2014 and 2021, had previously been the 'president of the global health division of UnitedHealth Group, a giant US private healthcare company'.[47] Stevens oversaw the government's 'five-year forward view'[48] and the 'Sustainability and Transformation Plans',[49] both of which have been heavily criticised by NHS campaigners for progressing the corporatisation agenda. And Stevens has now become Lord Simon Stevens, elevated in stature to the House of Lords for his efforts. Samantha Jones is not alone in Downing Street; she has been recently joined by someone called Bill Morgan, who is a private healthcare lobbyist with 'links to a series of controversial clients'.[50] The *Guardian* observed that Morgan had been hired to 'drive through NHS efficiencies'.

Things are ramping up fast under Rishi Sunak's leadership, with these appointments and with the recent formation of his NHS recovery taskforce, which appears to contain a number of Chief Executives of UK private healthcare companies. The tone of communication from senior politicians has changed rapidly. We're not told any more that the government wants to save the NHS. Therese Coffey, briefly Health Secretary in summer 2022, spoke openly about wanting to 'hold the NHS to account'. Steve Barclay, her successor, has declared that the NHS does not need any more money. And most illuminating of all, Sajid Javid (a former health minister himself) has contributed to an article in *The Times* newspaper where he stated that NHS patients should be charged for GP appointments and attendances at A&E. This is the most stark admission from a senior politician I have seen of a desire to entirely abandon the principles of the NHS, one of those principles, of course, being to provide a free health service at the point of use. After all, the public is already paying for the NHS through taxes. It is interesting that this statement came from a senior politician who has already declared he will not be running at the next election. One wonders whether it is this that has put him in a position to speak up, without fear of his political career lying in tatters at the public outcry. He will no doubt move on to other things; exciting opportunities perhaps, just like his predecessor Matt Hancock.

It is the presence, or absence, of a public outcry that will determine what comes next. This government is making it increasingly clear what its intentions are, in its closely drawn links with the private healthcare system, while it allows the public service to crumble. Our systems to hold the government to account are weak, and we cannot rely on the media or our traditional organisations to speak up, or the opposition, which is expressing a desire to involve privatisation within its future plans for the NHS too. But interestingly, and encouragingly, the public outcry has begun.

The most important thing you can do as a campaigner is to listen intently to what people are saying; gauge the current strength of feeling, the awareness about an issue, which parts people are knowledgeable about and where the gaps in information lie. It's the only way you can formulate an effective campaign; campaigning, after all, is about drawing together energy, harnessing it, and flinging it at a cause in the most powerful way possible, to yield a result. EveryDoctor began campaigning against the Health and Care Bill during the autumn months of 2021. And at that time, the campaigning was quite difficult, because we had to do a lot of explaining about what was going on, the background and the landscape. Many people weren't aware about the context, the NHS outsourcing into the private sector, the failed private contracts and the questionable links between politicians and the private healthcare sector in the UK.

In a campaign, the more time you spend explaining the cause itself, the less time and energy you have to lobby about the actual thing; in this case, the Bill that was moving through Parliament. It was tough, and ultimately, despite our efforts – the efforts of thousands upon thousands of people speaking up and demanding action from their MP, and other organisations working on similar campaigns too – we failed. The Bill went through Parliament. It has been enacted.

But now, after another 18 months of Westminster scandals, of suggestions of sleaze and corruption, the churn of Health Secretary after Health Secretary amid the chaos of this government (we have had five now, in the past five years), something has shifted. The public sees that the NHS isn't being taken care of. It sees that workers are struggling and aren't being supported, and that many of them, in health and in other sectors, are being pushed into going on strike because they have been poorly paid and poorly treated for so long.

So there is a backdrop now, a backdrop of discontent. And things are changing, rapidly. The media, which has not done enough, has not done enough for years to hold the government to account, is finally starting to ask questions. As the NHS reached the worst state it had ever been in, just after New Year 2023, I and many other NHS campaigners were invited onto media platforms, including the BBC, where pertinent questions were asked about the government's behaviour, about our proposals for solutions, about how we had got to this point. And there is the sense that there is a tipping point, an opportunity now.

When Sajid Javid wrote his piece in *The Times*, declaring that NHS patients should be charged for things that their taxes already pay for, there was an outcry like nothing I have seen before. It feels like a number of things have amalgamated and have caused the public to stop tolerating this situation. There have been times in the past, many times, when the public has stopped political trajectories and reversed decision-making. This can happen when the swell of public anger becomes loud enough. It feels as though the tide is turning on the politicians, and a tipping point has been reached for the NHS.

4

THE IMPACT

I met a lady recently at an event we were running about NHS privatisation. She had travelled a long distance to come and speak with us, and she walked into the lecture theatre with the aid of a walking stick. This lady, let's call her Joan, told me that she needed a knee replacement, and was in pain that was getting steadily worse all the time. She was getting very worried, because she had been told that patients on NHS waiting lists for knee replacements where she lived were over two years long. She had also been told that she had the option to join a local waiting list of her choosing, between several local hospitals, but that all of the waiting lists were equally long. Several people had suggested to her that she should 'go private'. But she explained to me that she had no money to pay for private healthcare. Joan didn't like to make a fuss, but she was finding things incredibly difficult, increasingly demanding. She was on a lot of painkillers, but these had side effects, and she was worried about taking too many, or having to take stronger ones as time went on.

CRITICAL

She described how waiting for her knee operation was affecting her whole life now; her mobility was impacted and she was finding it harder and harder to get around. She could no longer do some of the things she enjoyed, which was making her feel low. She felt anxious and scared, and incredibly let down by the NHS, which she had thought would care for her in her vulnerable moments. She had come along to our meeting to find out why this was happening. She didn't understand it; she'd paid her taxes all her life. Why wasn't the service working any more?

This lady is experiencing something that is now happening all over the country, to a growing number of people. Their everyday, commonplace health conditions and their inability to access the care they need is the real tragedy of what politicians have done to the NHS. The silent suffering of millions of people who should be able to access care, who were promised it, is a betrayal by politicians. This isn't a situation that is confined to patients awaiting knee surgery, or even surgery in general. The waiting times, delays and cancellations are affecting patients who need treatment for many different conditions, and their voices are not being sufficiently heard. At the end of the meeting, Joan came over to me and apologised for 'moaning', saying that there were probably people worse off than her, and that she probably shouldn't be complaining at all.

Situations like Joan's aren't often covered within the national press. We hear about the emergencies, but we don't hear about the commonplace operations and outpatient appointments that have been delayed or cancelled so many times as to cause a patient harm. We don't often read in the papers about the patients who are quietly suffering every day. One of the most concerning areas of increased patient waiting times is in mental health services, an area that is frequently neglected by politicians, despite repeated promises to improve things for patients. The *Independent* requested information from 48 NHS Trusts to find out the length of waiting lists and the availability of mental health beds for children in the NHS, and made this information public in January 2022.[1] The results revealed an enormous disparity in children's access to mental health services across the NHS. In some places, they were able to access specialist mental health support within seven days of a referral. But in six NHS Trusts there were children who had waited longer than a year for an assessment, and in one Trust a child had waited an extraordinary 1,019 days.

In order to have found their way onto an NHS waiting list for mental health assessment, these children will have been seen by another healthcare professional who established that they required support. That support is now lacking in so many cases, and this can have profound impacts not only on individual children, but on their families and support networks. It is a disaster, especially given the multiple claims in recent years from politicians including Theresa May,[2] David Cameron[3] and Matt Hancock[4] that mental health provision will be prioritised. Cameron even went so far as to promise a 'revolution' in mental health care. This promise was made in early 2016, and has not been realised by any of his political successors. Instead, things have become worse and worse.

CRITICAL

We know that prolonged waits for treatment can lead to worse health outcomes for patients, and for some people the impact of this will be very serious. This is one of the reasons we have treatment protocols for various conditions; very often, treatment is most effective if delivered within a specific time window. Such protocols are developed through the experiences of experts and using the evidence base available. It's why, for example, patients who are suspected to have sepsis are given their first dose of antibiotics quickly. Healthcare protocols help to keep patients safe.

The NHS is fortunate to have some of the most highly trained, competent healthcare professionals in the world, and the staff understand these protocols and do everything they can to stick to them. That's what the NHS targets are all about too; they afford a framework to provide efficient, timely care for patients. Waiting for treatment isn't just a matter of inconvenience. It can be the difference between life and death for some patients.

And this, I think, reveals the starkest impact that politicians' decisions have had upon the NHS. The service has been crippled to the point that the science cannot be adhered to. Healthcare professionals, researchers and scientists have made great strides in medicine during the twentieth and twenty-first centuries. Our knowledge base is so rich, and the UK has contributed to much of this; the NHS has been a part of this process of advancement and discovery over the past 75 years. We have experts and representative bodies who are knowledgeable about the best treatment available, the best techniques, and how best to apply this to save lives, to maximise quality of life, to maximise the health of our population.

But those experts, those bodies, with their rich knowledge base and expertise, have been largely disregarded by the government in recent years. As the situation in the NHS has deteriorated – waiting times lengthening, hospitals creaking under pressure, A&E departments experiencing overcrowding – many of the Royal Colleges have spoken up about their concerns regarding our failure to meet the targets. Eventually, after years of stating the facts and failing to be adequately listened to, the Academy of Medical Royal Colleges stated in a report in September 2022: 'the system is providing increasing proportions of care or services which are sub-standard, threaten patient safety, and should not be acceptable in a country with the resources that we have in the UK'.[5]

This is an extraordinary statement to have emanated from one of the most respected institutions in healthcare, and we would hope that its decision to speak up in such stark terms would yield results and push the government into action. Yet the report has not caused the reaction from the government that it should have done. The government failed, and continues to fail, to treat this situation with the gravity it deserves.

I speak to doctors every day about what is happening within the NHS, and what is concerning them the most at any given time. As things have deteriorated, more and more doctors are saying that they can no longer offer good care to their patients. I've heard doctors say that they'd be worried if their child, or parent, or friend ended up needing care from the service they work within.

They explain that the situation has deteriorated so significantly that care is being rationed within the service.
There is simply not enough to go around any more. And
while the newspapers might not be covering what's
happening to patients like Joan, which has made it hard
for the public to fully absorb what has been happening,
NHS staff are confronted with situations like hers day
in, day out. They have recognised that the situation is
worsening, and have been trying to raise the alarm in
various ways for a long time now.

NHS staff, after all, are the ones who have to explain
to patients that the waiting lists are long, or that the
operation they'd been patiently waiting for has been
cancelled again. They're the ones reassessing patients as
their symptoms deteriorate, perhaps as their analgesia
requirements have gone up. All the time knowing that if
only their patient could receive the operation, or proce-
dure, or treatment they need, their health would improve.
They are seeing the service unravel in its ability to meet
patients' needs in real time, every single day.

It's heart-wrenching for many clinicians, because they
are not able to provide the care which they would like to
offer their patients. GPs cannot refer a patient to a
specialist and feel safe in the knowledge that that patient
will receive specialist input in a timely manner. A patient
will be scheduled for an operation but may wait endlessly
on a list for their turn. And as ever more patients are
blocked from accessing what they need, many are coming
to harm within a healthcare system that is broken, in
collapse, in freefall. This, ultimately, is the impact of politicians' decisions and their actions upon the NHS. The

creation of a system that is no longer inclusionary in nature, providing comprehensive healthcare, but rather exclusionary, giving less care to fewer people, and worsening all the time.

The situation is terrible for patients, devastating in many cases. And it is also terrible for NHS staff. Over the past few decades, as politicians have made stepwise reforms, exacerbated by the relentless 'austerity' cuts of the 2010s, the staff have had to absorb these upheavals, enact the changes, and keep patients safe in a system that has been restructured again and again. At best, these changes have felt like arduous exercises in PR for one new government or another, trying to stamp its mark on the NHS. At worse, the reforms have caused chaos and cutbacks, the loss of staff members and a degradation in the service that staff are able to provide. Staff cuts. Service cuts. Bed cuts.

And for the most part, NHS staff just got on with it through all of these changes, doing the best they could for their patients. But things have changed now. You can't keep reforming a thing – cutting bits, losing staff and failing to invest – and expect it to keep functioning. Staff became more frustrated, and more vocal, and more concerned. It didn't happen quickly, but over a number of years it became apparent to many NHS staff that the service was deteriorating and that politicians were not stepping in to rectify the situation, reverse poor policy and improve things.

As we got to the end of the 2010s, it felt like there was a growing disconnect between the behaviour of the government, which seemed to be undermining the service in any way it could, and the staff, who were desperately trying to hold the service together under more and more pressure. But when the pandemic hit, things worsened still further for NHS staff. It opened up a great chasm in the differences in attitude and behaviour displayed by them and the government.

This government failed to protect staff adequately, failed to listen to their concerns, and largely failed to support them through the most significant public health crisis the NHS has ever absorbed, while the staff shouldered the responsibility for the safety of the public. The EveryDoctor team was in close communication with a large number of frontline doctors throughout the pandemic, gathering up-to-date information in order to support and advocate for NHS workers and their patients. The first issue that came to light was the lack of safe PPE being provided for many UK healthcare workers.

PPE was in short supply because of poor planning by the UK government, despite having run a simulation exercise called Exercise Cygnus in 2016 to explore the UK's readiness to tackle a similar threat to COVID-19.[6] We were able to piece together information about the types of PPE that were available to clinicians in the early days of the pandemic. While doctors working within intensive care units were generally being provided with safe PPE, many of the NHS staff working in community settings were not prioritised. We heard about doctors who were sent a single box of gloves for a GP practice with 50 members of staff, along with one box of single-use flimsy blue surgical masks. GPs had to go to hardware stores, and fashion PPE out of whatever was available. Some of the PPE that was sent to GPs was even out of date, and had new 'use by stickers' stuck over the top of the old ones, which looked like it had been intentionally done. Doctors were terrified, and yet carried on going to work to do whatever they could to keep their patients safe.

Certain memories stand out. I remember being sent a photograph of one GP's family standing at a dining table making visors out of Perspex sheets in a makeshift production line. I remember a photo of one of our GP members, inadequately protected in a plastic apron as she drove out to home visits for her sickest patients at the height of the crisis. Doctors within our network shared information about what they were doing; fashioning PPE from whatever came to hand; sanitary towels stuck to plastic laminator sheets to make visors, Perspex sheets bought in local hardware stores.

People were having to go through old cupboards in offices in NHS hospitals and were using whatever they found, ordering things off the internet, or relying on kind people local to them who had a 3D printer or ran the design technology department in a school to help create some of the makeshift equipment. Anything really. There were alarming stories of staff with nothing else to hand in the early days, wrapping cling film around their noses and mouths as they attended to patients. Heroic stories of consultants putting padlocks on operating theatre doors and refusing to take the lock off until safe PPE was found by hospital management. And desperate, tragic situations, where staff, despite not having adequate PPE, were instructed to continue caring for patients who were sick with COVID-19, and in doing so, became sick themselves and died. Many staff died; by January 2021, the ONS stated that 883 health and social care staff had lost their lives in the UK.[7]

Healthcare workers spoke up, and members of the public spoke up with them, trying to find out what was happening, get some clear answers from the government and some assurances about when the situation would improve. But the information being shared with staff was patchy and incomplete, and quite often as developments occurred throughout the pandemic, they would only find out about it when reading an announcement in the media. That's no way to treat staff managing the frontline of a national crisis. They deserved to know what was going on. When it became apparent that GP surgeries weren't receiving what they needed in mid-March 2020, EveryDoctor printed a placard outlining our demands, went to the headquarters of NHS England and invited a national television crew down, in order to exert pressure on the decision-makers, who we felt were withholding important information. We were interviewed on the national news and received a call within several hours promising us that PPE was on its way to many NHS facilities. At the time, I felt reassured. In retrospect, I think the person who gave me that information exaggerated how organised their team was, how much PPE was being sent out, and vastly minimised the severity of the situation.

Soon, even the doctors working in the intensive care units started to struggle with supply. On 18 April 2020, the *Guardian* reported the words of Robert Jenrick, the Housing, Communities and Local Government secretary, who had spoken about this at the government's Saturday press conference. He said: 'supply in some areas, particularly gowns and certain types of masks and aprons, is in short supply at the moment, and that must be an extremely anxious time for people working on the frontline, but they should be assured that we are doing everything we can to correct this issue, and to get them the equipment that they need'.[8] Unsurprisingly, this did not reassure frontline workers. They were still expected to go to work, regardless of these failures.

The PPE situation was not the only area where the government failed to listen and respond to concerns from the staff. We constructed a campaign called #ProtectNHSWorkers, detailing five areas that needed immediate policy changes, including providing a death-in-service benefit for the families of staff members who had tragically died, and providing sick pay for temporary staff who were becoming unwell with the virus. We did win some concessions and support for staff, not least the death-in-service benefits that we and others campaigned for, and changes to the PPE policy. But the protections that were won for workers were only achieved through the immense pushback of thousands upon thousands of people, along with politicians we were working with to press for these measures. Nothing was won easily. It felt, all the way through the pandemic, as if the government was doing the absolute minimum to support NHS staff, while maximising the press opportunities to make itself look good.

Staff had mixed emotions and differing opinions about the 'clap for carers' initiative, largely because it was adopted by a government that was failing to support them in so many ways. Some pervasive descriptions and imagery became associated with healthcare workers during the pandemic that became problematic for healthcare workers. As reported at the end of April 2020: 'A Hull nursing expert insists calling healthcare staff heroes and angels during the coronavirus outbreak is "unhelpful" and says having the right protective equipment is what they need.'[9]

Many of these descriptions were being used by members of the public, who were very supportive of the staff and the service, and the doctors in our network really valued their support. But some of these images suggested that healthcare workers were different to other people, imbued with special qualities of strength, nobility and courage, which meant that they weren't seen as simply workers, needing the same support and protections as other people. Such an idea is unhelpful at any time, not just in the middle of a pandemic, suggesting that healthcare workers can handle longer hours than other people, or can tolerate being overworked. These images of heroism can also infer that if a healthcare worker is 'truly dedicated' to their profession, they won't require proper pay.

Because the government wasn't supporting staff properly, because it took for granted the enormous sacrifices that were being made and didn't treat them with respect, many staff began to feel like a commodity. Especially so as the government asked more and more from them as the pandemic went on and the situation developed. The COVID-19 vaccination programme in England, which has been hailed multiple times as a great triumph by our government, was actually a success in large part because of the astronomical effort of GPs and volunteers. As mentioned earlier, GPs in England were asked, in the run-up to Christmas 2020, to set up the first COVID-19 vaccine centres, and had to plan these centres at extremely short notice. They were not offered any upfront funding to find staff to help, but despite immense pressures and challenges, they succeeded. It was their efforts in this regard that propelled us into such a successful start to the COVID-19 vaccination programme.

GPs did this alongside caring for their patients as normal. Despite much misinformation to the contrary, they have cared for their patients all the way through the pandemic. They have been on the frontline of this emergency just like all other frontline workers, and in part because they were inadequately protected, many GPs have died of COVID-19. At the beginning of the pandemic, they were asked to move to telephone consultations for the majority of their patients. As the *Guardian* reported on 6 March 2020: 'In a significant policy change, NHS bosses want England's 7,000 GP surgeries to start conducting as many remote consultations as soon as possible, replacing patient visits with phone, video, online or text contact.'[10] It was GPs, in many cases, who pushed back against this policy and maintained face-to-face contact with many of their patients, all the way through the pandemic, wherever they felt that it was in the interests of patients to do this.

Some patients are happier with telephone consultations; these can be quicker and easier for them than a trip to the GP surgery, and during the pandemic many were reluctant to leave their houses for fear of catching COVID-19. I spoke to GPs throughout the pandemic, and I have yet to encounter a single one who moved entirely to telephone consultations. This policy, however, devised by NHS England and only followed in part by GPs, who prioritised the safety and well-being of their patients, has been used as a weapon to demonise GPs in the national press. This is where the treatment of NHS staff becomes truly appalling. Despite all of their sacrifices, everything they have done to keep the public safe, as we emerged from the pandemic some media outlets began what has felt like a sustained campaign against GPs, and one that received support from the then Health Secretary, Sajid Javid.

The *Daily Mail* started what it called the 'Let's See GPs Face to Face campaign', which began in May 2021,[11] and this ramped up during the autumn. A number of articles published in national media outlets misrepresented the situation regarding telephone consultations, and maligned GPs, including a scathing piece in *The Spectator* from September 2021 headed: 'It's time for GPs to stop hiding behind their telephones'.[12] The *Daily Mail* heralded in October: 'The new face-to-face revolution: Sajid Javid launches overhaul in GP access so all patients can see a doctor in person ... with league tables and "hit squads" for those that fail'. It declared that 'The nine-point plan is a major victory for the Daily Mail's Let's See GPs Face to Face campaign.'[13]

Throughout this period, I was speaking to NHS GPs on a daily basis, and they were horrified to have their work described in this way. Throughout, they were offering patients the safest and most appropriate care they could, while under extreme pressure. Many GPs I spoke to felt that abuse from patients was getting worse, specifically because of things that they had read in the papers. I heard about patients being so aggressive that, in one practice, the reception staff at a GP surgery all had to leave. Another had a door kicked in by a patient who was frustrated that his medication wasn't available (he had, in fact, gone to the wrong GP surgery to collect his prescription). The abuse escalated to such an extent that some surgeries reported they were having to 'man the front desk' solely with clinical staff, because the administrative staff didn't feel able to explain why the service was under such pressure and couldn't cope with the rising tide of abuse.

A group of medical leaders wrote a joint statement to the government, which the *Guardian* covered in October 2021, stating: 'they are urging ministers to be "honest and transparent" about the intense strain on the NHS after a spike in threats and assaults on frontline staff'. The paper also said: 'it comes amid a growing belief among senior doctors that ministers' insistence that GPs should offer face-to-face appointments, that hospitals need to improve waiting times as soon as possible, and that managers of "failing" hospitals with persistently long delays for care could be sacked are all part of a deliberate government strategy to try to blame the NHS for its many problems'.[14] The concerted effort to scapegoat staff has been deeply disturbing. Javid went so far as to state in the House of Commons that 'more GPs should be offering face-to-face access', and that 'we intend to do a lot more about it'.[15]

Just days later, a patient attacked a GP and other practice staff in Manchester in a surgery waiting room, resulting in the GP sustaining a skull fracture and other staff members also sustaining injuries. In coverage of the incident, it was stated: 'medics in Greater Manchester suggested recent criticism of GPs in the media is fuelling abuse'.[16] This feeling was widespread throughout our network of doctors. The government should have been doing everything to support staff at such a difficult time, instead of blaming them for problems.

One might wonder what the motive would be, to scapegoat staff at such a pressured time for the health service. Cynically, one might suspect it could have had something to do with advancing the Health and Care Act 2022,[17] the controversial legislation that has further fragmented the NHS in England, and has increased the powers of the Secretary of State for Health and Social Care to intervene in local healthcare decision-making. By deflecting negative attention onto GPs at such a pressured time, politicians perhaps avoided some of the scrutiny they would have received for this Bill. However, the abuse did not stop when the Bill received Royal Assent and was implemented, and, horribly, it seems likely that this scapegoating of NHS GPs is part of a wider trend, denigrating NHS staff in a bid to deflect or divert attention from the government's own failings towards the NHS.

Staff have been treated terribly by this government; taken advantage of, misrepresented, underpaid, and starved of the support they have desperately needed during the worst crisis the NHS has ever faced. The situation continues to worsen. We are now facing a situation where we are missing almost 10 per cent of the entire NHS staff workforce in England,[18] and it's no surprise that staff are leaving in droves. There have been significant real-terms pay cuts across the healthcare sector, with (probably the starkest example) NHS consultant pay dropping by 34.9 per cent in real terms since 2008/09.[19] Nurses' salaries have also fallen significantly, by an average of 8 per cent since 2010.[20] And they were poorly paid even in 2010, their incredible skill and expertise undervalued, so their pay has dropped from a much lower starting point. The situation is appalling. Many nurses and other NHS staff are paid so poorly now that they are forced to rely on food banks. Over a quarter (27 per cent) of NHS Trusts in England now run their own food banks for staff, and as reported by the *Guardian* in September 2022, 19 per cent more plan to open one. The *Guardian* goes on to state: 'Lack of money is also prompting some NHS staff to call in sick in the days before they get paid because they can no longer afford the travel costs for their shift.'[21] Others are taking a second job outside the NHS in an effort to make ends meet. It's a shocking state of affairs.

The NHS pensions crisis is ongoing, with senior doctors cutting their hours because they simply can't afford the tax bills they are being hit with. We hear from our network of doctors that it is incredibly difficult for many staff to switch off even when they're not at work, because they are continually telephoned or emailed by their workplaces to ask if they can do another shift, another weekend on call. And as the staff numbers drop – doctors and nurses feeling pushed out of professions they studied and trained hard for, many seeking other jobs, or leaving the country, or taking early retirement – the situation becomes even more stressful for those who remain. I hear regularly from doctors who would like to leave their jobs but are staying purely out of a sense of loyalty to their colleagues, who they don't want to abandon.

It came as no surprise when a health select committee inquiry was published in June 2021 that revealed widespread burnout across NHS staff. As the *BMJ* reported at the time,[22] the evidence given to MPs spoke of 'feelings of low energy or exhaustion, increased mental distance from or negative feelings about the job, and reduced professional effectiveness'. It went on to state: 'Jeremy Hunt, committee chair, said, "Workforce burnout across the NHS and care systems now presents an extraordinarily dangerous risk to the future functioning of both services."' Many staff are simply unable to endure any more, and are leaving. The *Observer* reported in February 2022 that in the preceding year, 400 NHS staff members had left their jobs in England every single week.[23] This isn't the career many people thought they were entering into. Healthcare workers pursue their careers to help people.

The workforce have been trying to hold the service together for years despite the actions of this government. Many staff are leaving their jobs within the NHS now, because they feel unable to continue working within a service that takes so much from them, with their own mental health often deteriorating as a result. The moral injury, stress and trauma that has been loaded upon many staff members is absolutely appalling. I receive messages regularly from doctors who say their personal lives have been deeply affected by the strains of their job, who have been diagnosed with mental health conditions. Some have even experienced suicidal thoughts because of the stress and the ever-present realisation that they are not doing enough, cannot do enough, for patients who are being failed within this collapsing system.

Staff have been expected to absorb more and more as time has gone on, and the government has not displayed any compassion or remorse for this. They have been commodified and treated horrendously. And it is not just the staff who have been treated in this way. In recent years, other elements of the service have been commodified too, mined for profit or value. An example is the way this government has managed NHS land. The Naylor Review was a report written in 2017, after being commissioned by the then Health Secretary Jeremy Hunt. The idea was to 'develop a new estate strategy'.[24] The 'estate' is all of the land and the buildings that are owned by the NHS, and it's a huge amount of land, because clinical facilities take up a lot of space. It comprises many very valuable bits of property, especially when hospitals are in city centres.

There was enormous concern when the Naylor Review was first announced (and then endorsed by Theresa May[25]), because of concerns about selling off public assets to plug a funding hole created by the Conservative government. There were also worries among campaigners and many politicians that some of the plots that had been put up for sale were in fact still being used as NHS facilities. Despite a huge amount of press coverage at the time of the review's publication, there has been remarkably little recent media attention given to what has happened in terms of the amount of land sold off. NHS Digital produces a quarterly report, described as the 'surplus land' report, which details the land for sale and the land sold,[26] but it's not a subject that receives very much scrutiny or discussion, and this should probably change. There are important questions that should be asked about the sale of NHS land; after all, land tends to go up in value. If we sell off these assets now, it is unlikely that future governments will be able to afford to buy large plots of land to enable hospital building projects.

As well as the bricks and mortar and the very land that the NHS operates on, there is the issue of patient data. There have been growing concerns in recent years about the data that the NHS holds on all of us, which for many private companies is seen as an untapped source of income. It raises all kinds of ethical questions about privacy and consent. The *Financial Times* conducted an analysis in 2021 of the NHS Digital Data Release Register over the past five years. And in its reporting, it stated that the analysis 'raises concerns over potential conflicts of interests and a lack of transparency about what happens to the data after it is shared'.[27] It explained that most of those accessing the data do so for planning and research purposes, and are organisations such as councils and universities. But 13 per cent of the total number of recipients were commercial organisations, including pharmaceutical companies. As described by the *Financial Times*: 'Critics argue that patients are often unaware of the NHS's data-sharing practices, and even if they withhold consent it can be difficult to prevent their data from being disseminated externally. While the NHS provides a "national data opt-out" option for patients, it still shared full, pseudonymised data sets with external organisations in 84 percent of instances when opt-outs had been exercised.'

It is a problem that is taking on more significance for people, as the value of so-called 'big data' is being increasingly realised, and considered an asset. In 2021, a scheme called the 'General Practice Data for Planning and Research' was delayed to September and then put on hold altogether, after a campaign led to more than a million people opting out of their data being shared. Campaigners medConfidential were very critical of the scheme. Phil Booth, the coordinator of medConfidential, said in an article for the *Observer* that NHS Digital (which was running the scheme) 'made a bunch of public promises and we very much want to see how those promises are delivered. We've always said there are fairly legitimate, ethical, research and planning uses that can be made of this data – it just has to be done right. The question is, what's going on behind closed doors right now in terms of people lobbying against those [concessions] or for particular exceptions to them.'[28]

The debate concerning the value of public data within research, versus individuals' right to protect their own data, is a very important one. It deserves a public conversation to determine a right course of action. This government attempted to push through a change despite concerns about safety and transparency, simply offering an opt-out for people who didn't want to be involved. Many patients would simply not have known about the scheme and therefore been unable to opt out. And more broadly, one of the developments following campaigners' work was for NHS Digital to say that they 'will continue working with patients, clinicians, researchers and charities to inform further safeguards'.[29] This statement alone is alarming; one would hope that the scheme already incorporated robust safeguards by the time it was in the active planning stages.

And so the impacts of this government upon the NHS are laid bare. Decisions upon decisions that have stacked up for years, weakening the service through cutback after cutback, and then failing to respond when things worsened, at first incrementally and then in an accelerating crisis, as we transition from devastating pandemic to the devastation of care-rationing and millions of people unable to access the treatment they require. Treating the staff as commodities and failing to support them in their work, and creating a situation where our skilled staff are now leaving in droves. Finding new ways to mine the system for value, instead of shoring up the service and ensuring its future sustainability.

The inaction of senior politicians during the pandemic received sympathy from some quarters: from those who felt they were doing their best in extreme circumstances, and that things were simply moving too fast for them to respond quickly enough to all of the problems. That sympathy does not hold now; the situation has worsened

month after month after month and this government has
not taken the action required to improve things for the
patients, and the staff. They could have fixed the cumber-
some pension rules. They could be paying staff better.
They could be investing money into the crumbling buildings. And instead they have repeatedly siphoned off large
sums into buying up capacity in private hospitals, into
paying management consultancy organisations enormous amounts of money, and they have pushed through
a Bill that we fear will make the situation even worse,
and fragment the service still further through the creation of yet more outsourced short-term contracts.

The impacts of their betrayal are being felt in all areas
of the NHS now. GP surgeries, community services,
ambulances, hospitals are all under enormous pressure.
The government has claimed for many years now that it
intends to 'fix' the social care crisis.[30] But it hasn't happened,
and the result is a situation where in some hospitals in
England, up to one in three patients in hospital beds
are well enough to be discharged from hospital, but
have nowhere to go. The flow of patients through a
hospital is affected by this. A&E staff cannot admit
patients from A&E into hospital wards as quickly as they
would like to, meaning that A&E departments are
becoming extremely crowded. Ambulance bays fill up,
with paramedics hoping to hand over their patients to
A&E staff, but unable to do so, often for hours at a time.
And all of this means that there are fewer ambulances on
the roads, available to pick up the next patient who
needs emergency help. Ambulance waiting times are
routinely missing the safety standards that have been set.

When a patient needs emergency treatment – if, for example, they have suffered a severe fall or have symptoms that indicate they could be having a heart attack or stroke – it is imperative that they can access healthcare quickly and safely. This, after all, is what the NHS promises to do. And this is what the government has been entrusted to provide for the public. Politicians, this particular government, have been given endless policy suggestions and advice from many healthcare leaders, and much of this has been ignored. There are measures that would have alleviated the situation and made people safer. For instance, if the government had chosen to pay NHS staff better, it would have improved the recruitment and retention of highly skilled workers, helping to avoid the current huge staffing gaps.

The situation that the politicians have created, the inability of millions of people to access the care they need and that they are promised, is now forcing many to use private healthcare. A report from Engage Britain, which the *Guardian* reported on in September 2022, showed that 10 per cent of all UK adults had turned to the private sector in the previous 12 months, and 'of those, almost two-thirds (63 per cent) did so because they faced long delays or could not access treatment on the NHS'.[31] At the moment, around 13 per cent of Britons have medical insurance.[32] It's likely that this figure will rise, given the current situation. But even if we set aside for a minute the fact that the NHS is a public service paid for by taxes, and that it is very wrong that the public should be forced into using private healthcare due to its demise, the private sector itself does not have the capacity to absorb the current burden of illness among UK citizens.

There is a pervasive myth among some politicians that the private healthcare sector in the UK is huge, and consists of an army of healthcare workers. But there is simply no truth in this. The BMA put out a medical staffing report in July 2021, which on the topic of doctors working in the private sector states: 'given they currently draw largely on the same pool of doctors, workforce planning assessments must acknowledge the fact that many of the doctors working in private hospitals are also NHS doctors'.[33]

The BMA sought to find out how many doctors were working within the private sector in the UK, and has stated that available information for England indicate that '860 FTE (full-time equivalent) doctors were employed by independent health providers in 2020 compared to 486 FTE doctors in September 2015 – a 77% increase over 5 years'. In contrast, the report stated that the NHS employs 159,100 doctors (including all secondary care doctors who work in hospitals, and all GPs). The 860 doctors employed within the independent sector doesn't tell the full story, because some NHS doctors do some part-time work within the private sector on top of their NHS work.[34] And this rise in numbers of doctors exclusively working within the independent sector is notable for its growth. However, two things are clear. First, the number of doctors employed by private companies is absolutely dwarfed by those working within the NHS, and so their ability to swoop in and save the NHS is minimal, and second, if the private sector seeks to expand its provision of healthcare to support the NHS, it will probably be poaching NHS doctors' time in order to do so.

And so, even if large numbers of patients who are currently on NHS waiting lists chose to spend their money on paying for private healthcare in the near future, the likelihood is that the private sector itself would soon reach saturation point and be unable to deliver the healthcare required, given that NHS waiting lists are the longest they have ever been in the service's history. And, of course, lots of people cannot afford to turn to the private sector in a vulnerable moment anyway, particularly at the moment, during a national crisis in which a huge number of people are struggling to pay their bills and heat their homes.

And so this situation, worsening every single month, is creating a two-tier healthcare system that is becoming more entrenched month on month, as the waiting lists get progressively longer, and more people are denied access to the care they need. Neither of the largest political parties are currently putting forward viable solutions to the crisis. At the time of writing, in early 2023, Rishi Sunak has recently held an 'NHS forum' to discuss the crisis. He invited 'representatives from the public and private sectors'[35] to the meeting, including many NHS leaders. But the outcomes, which include plans for 'diagnostic hubs' and 'virtual wards', are unlikely to be implemented at the speed or scale required to really tackle the situation head-on. And, judging from the feedback of lots of doctors within our network who have been discussing this, the solutions put forward will put the onus on current staff to do even more work. We're in the middle of an extraordinary crisis; we need more radical ideas than this. The situation needs to be treated as an emergency, not one requiring a solution in the medium to long term, heaping yet more pressure upon staff who are already struggling to cope under unbelievable demands. The best way to approach this crisis would be to support staff: pay them properly, reward them for doing extra hours, sort out their pensions, and provide them with adequate mental health support. The NHS's ability to cope with all of this comes down to its staff.

Labour hasn't been challenging the government adequately on immediate solutions that need to be found, but instead has been focused on its manifesto for the next general election. It is putting forward a plan to drive down waiting lists by turning to the private sector.[36] As mentioned above, the private sector is unlikely to have the necessary capacity to achieve this goal. And even if the UK private healthcare sector was sufficiently large and robust to have the capacity to provide the support that Streeting and Starmer hope for, this isn't a sustainable plan that will strengthen the NHS for the future. It's a short-term plan to patch things up and will be effected at enormous cost to the taxpayer.

In short, neither of our major political parties is coming up with a plan that properly invests in the NHS's future, that strengthens the service for the long term and focuses squarely on the three principles that underpin the service. It would be much more challenging, of course, to invest in the NHS and properly build up the service to offer comprehensive healthcare, free to all at the point of use, with equal access for all. But this is ultimately what the public wants. Many public polls have been run into various aspects of the NHS, and the public's opinion of the service. And the polls consistently show that the public wants the service to continue. One such example is the Survation poll that was run in 2020 for the think-tank We Own It. The results showed that 76 per cent of the public wanted the NHS to be 'reinstated as a fully public service' and only 15 per cent of respondents wanted the NHS to have the continued involvement of private companies.[37]

There is the sense, now, that the public is waking up to the impacts of everything the politicians have done, continue to do, and wish to do in the future. Twenty years ago, ten, five even, campaigners would talk about the future impact of what the politicians were doing, but it wasn't palpable to everyone because they weren't struggling to access healthcare themselves. When campaigners raised concerns about privatisation, about the outsourcing of NHS services to be run by private companies, or talked about the impact of the PFI debt, many people struggled to understand the concerns. I wasn't aware of the implications myself until about six or seven years ago. And I was working within the service myself, witnessing the situation day in and day out.

But things are different now. You can sense, speaking to people online, that the public mood is changing, that large numbers are waking up to the impacts of politicians upon the NHS. Even if a person isn't on an NHS waiting list themselves, or hasn't recently experienced a very long wait at an A&E department, the chances are they'll know someone who has. A friend or a relative, a loved one who is struggling to access the care they need. And this has an impact on people. What the politicians have not accounted for is how it feels to be unable to access healthcare. It weighs on people's minds, it worries them, it is frustrating and terrifying, it causes huge anxiety. People are living with symptoms that haven't been explained to them, pain that isn't being properly alleviated. And for many, they're getting worse and they're not getting any answers.

All this is layered on top of other problems they're having; other problems that leave them feeling unsupported within our society. There have been significant cuts to school budgets, which is impacting on the experience that children, parents and teachers have in our schools. There is an energy crisis and the government has failed to do enough to support many of the most vulnerable people in our communities, many suffering greatly as a result. A woman recently died after being admitted to hospital with hypothermia and a chest infection. ITV reported that 'hospital notes indicate her illness was linked to the fact she could not afford to put her heating on'.[38] It is devastating that this has come to pass, and it is very unlikely that this lady's death was or will be an isolated incident.

This government has utilised various tactics to ascribe blame to others, to divide and conquer between staff and patients; for example, in its treatment of GPs, or, earlier, of junior doctors during our contract dispute in 2016. At times this has worked, because of the power of various media outlets and their campaigns waged in relation to particular staff groups. But there is the sense that in this, too, the public mood is changing. There is a wave of strikes occurring across many sectors currently; numerous disputes involving workers in different UK industries: rail, postal workers, nurses, teachers, ambulance drivers, and others too (junior doctors are being balloted to strike as I write this).

NHS staff have had enough. When healthcare workers contemplate striking, demanding better conditions and the pay rise they deserve, patient safety is a driving factor in why they are choosing to do this. They are fighting for staff to be supported, for the workforce to be valued and for the future of the NHS to be protected. And as reports mount up of their colleagues leaving, of them having to take on unbelievable numbers of shifts just to make ends meet, of needing to use food banks or being unable to afford the bus fare to get to work, the public is increasingly listening. It's scary to consider that, in your time of need, you might be cared for by someone who is exhausted after working for too many hours. The public understands that staff should be supported and well rested. It's not all about the pay. It's about safety for patients too.

And despite intense efforts from the government to malign these workers and accuse them of irresponsibility and of causing problems for the public, NHS workers are currently looking robust, and public support for their efforts is strong. The *Telegraph* reported in January 2023[39] that public support for striking health workers had actually increased compared to four weeks previously.

THE IMPACT

The tide is turning, and finally people are seeing the impacts of politicians' decisions – decisions that were not taken with the welfare of patients in mind, nor with the sustainability of the service in mind, nor with the three core principles of the NHS in mind.

Neither of the major political parties has realised the strength of this feeling yet, the weight of public opinion that I suspect will come crashing down and force them into action. For too long now, politicians have got away with what they've done. But public concern is palpable on social media, in the emails EveryDoctor is receiving, in the messages I receive from doctors every day. There is a tide of energy building, and it is difficult to see why it would dissipate now, with the situation worsening month after month after month. People have finally had enough, and I suspect they're about to start pushing back en masse.

5

THE SOLUTION

The situation in the NHS cannot continue like this; things are deteriorating all the time. We can track the deterioration through the monthly statistics, which reveal just how badly the NHS is failing on its targets; how long it is taking ambulances to reach patients who are experiencing life-threatening emergencies now; how many people each month wait for more than 12 hours to be admitted to a hospital ward after they've been assessed in A&E; what proportion of patients are treated within A&E within the four-hour target. And then there's the waiting lists of course, which are extraordinarily long. The government has said in early 2023 that waiting lists are a top priority, but we're yet to see any meaningful change. And beyond the numbers, the statistics, there are people. Every one of those numbers represents a patient who is being failed; so many cannot access what they need from the NHS in a timely manner because of the decisions of politicians.

This is awful to contemplate, and it is equally awful to realise the impact of all this on staff. They still continue to go to work day after day, attempting to keep patients as safe as they can, often in impossible circumstances, without adequate support. The NHS wasn't meant to be like this, it shouldn't be like this. Thankfully, people are becoming more aware of the situation all the time. So we have an opportunity to push back. But we'll need to get organised, be clear about what we want to change, and mobilise an enormous number of people to speak up. There's no time to lose.

Our primary concern, of course, comes down to demand, and the inability of the NHS to currently cope with the healthcare needs of the population. The health service needs to be invested in, strengthened, to meet the needs of the public. But our concerns also relate to the way the system has been restructured over decades by politicians; the current existence of many private health-care companies running NHS services all over England. Because it looks as though NHS campaigners have been correct for years: the infiltration of private companies has now been linked to a negative impact on patient care. In June 2022, a study came out in one of the most respected medical publications in the world, *The Lancet*. The study – an observational one and the first of its kind – had focused on NHS services being run by private healthcare companies between 2013 and 2020. It found that 'the privatisation of NHS services in England over the past seven years has been linked to a decline in the quality of patient care'.[1] It also identified that increased rates of private outsourcing were associated with 'signif-icantly increased rates of treatable mortality'.[2] In other words, private outsourcing within the NHS was linked to deaths that could have been avoidable with effective healthcare.

This study was given widespread coverage in the UK national press and beyond[3] for a day or two, and among the medical community it caused considerable consternation. But it hasn't resulted in the kind of shock, or action, that we might have expected from politicians. In fact, the Health and Care Act 2022, which many NHS campaigners fear will enable even more private outsourcing to infiltrate the NHS, was implemented several weeks after this study came out. This situation needs to end now. We must demand that the NHS is brought fully back into public ownership, and stop the private outsourcing of NHS services.

And if we hope to push back effectively and change things, we must also keep a close eye on what is happening, what politicians and a largely complicit UK media are saying, and what they are likely to be planning next. Unbelievably, even amid the current crisis, politicians are beginning conversations suggesting they wish to disregard one of the NHS's principles entirely, and begin to charge patients within certain services. If we are to successfully stop this trajectory of NHS destruction and turn things around, we need to pay attention to their next moves as well as repair the damage that has been done to our public healthcare service.

Changes to the NHS are not implemented out of the blue. Tentative suggestions are introduced into the public discourse, 'think pieces' are written in the media, politicians start making public suggestions about policy aimed at testing the water, initiating conversations and influencing public thinking around the NHS (and a number of other issues within UK politics of course). A spate of articles appeared in certain UK media outlets in 2022 about how the public had 'fallen out of love with the NHS',[4] after a poll showed that satisfaction levels with the service had dropped. These articles were cleverly written, the thrust of each being that because patients were currently unhappy with the service they were receiving, they no longer valued the NHS as a service.

At around the same time, a new suggestion emerged: that perhaps the UK should adopt the practices of healthcare systems from other countries, because our own health service was inefficient. Politicians and the media are incredibly adept at seeding curiosity about certain ideas, and this idea is being shared more and more frequently now. I notice that particularly on Twitter, people are asking about this, which is usually a telling sign that an idea is gaining momentum.

I was troubled to see this suggestion legitimised when the BBC published a piece on 24 September 2022, entitled 'Can the NHS learn from Germany's health system?' The piece was extremely positive in its description of insurance-based healthcare, explaining that in Germany, 'people can choose which fund they sign up to. These are paid for by deductions from wages with employee and employer contributions. Some small out-of-pocket payments are required for hospital visits and medicines.'[5] The piece chose to focus on the recent lowering of public satisfaction with the NHS from opinion polls, but not the results of opinion polls that consistently show the public's support for the NHS.

There was also no mention in the piece about why the NHS existed in the first place, or the principles it is based upon. And despite this article featuring several comments from leaders at the King's Fund and the Nuffield Trust, neither organisation chose to mention the historical efficiency of the NHS, nor its value to the British public. Instead, they commented on the potential costs of setting up an insurance-based system, or the administrative costs of such a system.

The BBC's piece even went so far as to feature comments from the right-wing think-tank the Institute of Economic Affairs, which describes itself as 'the UK's original free-market think-tank.[6] The piece stated that 'Dr Kristian Niemietz, of the Institute of Economic Affairs, thinks it could be a blueprint for reform in the UK: "Social health insurance systems tend to have better healthcare outcomes. Patients enjoy a greater degree of individual choice and benefit from shorter waiting times. Switching to a social health insurance system would not be a panacea. But if we want to combine the best aspects of a public system with the best aspects of a consumer-focused market-driven system, social health insurance is a tried and tested way to do that."'[7]

Conversations around charging within the NHS aren't new. The Conservative government took steps to scrutinise those accessing NHS healthcare some years ago. As the campaign group Docs not Cops explains on its website, 'on Monday 23rd October 2017, NHS England introduced regulations requiring ID checks for all patients accessing most secondary (non-emergency) care. This includes but (is) not limited to maternity/ante-natal care, paediatrics (children) and cancer treatment. Trusts are forced to charge upfront those who cannot provide ID to prove their eligibility for NHS treatment. These regulations follow the introduction of a Health Surcharge – paid on top of Visa application fees.'[8]

But the conversations are gathering pace and becoming more prominent. Most recently we have seen senior politicians directly stating that they would like to see changes involving patients paying for services. Rishi Sunak, with his pledge (currently on hold) to charge patients for missed NHS appointments. And Sajid Javid, who has stated in a piece in *The Times* that he thinks NHS patients should be paying for GP appointments and A&E attendances. Their rhetoric is ramping up. If the politicians get away with charging patients in this way, just as they have got away with numerous previous reforms that have pulled the NHS away from its original principles, it will mark a total breakaway from the NHS constitution. NHS privatisation will go beyond the outsourcing of services, the buying up of GP practices and the selling off of NHS buildings. It would truly spell the end for the NHS as we know it.

The government is clever with its messaging, and its strategy. It holds enormous power through its ability to communicate with the public through the media, and it is seeking to capitalise on a crisis of its own making, to destroy a public service that does not belong to it. It belongs to the public. And I have learned, through the campaigning I have done over the past seven years, that it is very difficult to oppose what the government is doing. Its own communications machinery is strategically run and has a great deal of money behind it; it is able to run expensive political ads across social media, for example, and politicians regularly dismiss concerns and even attack the campaigners who are attempting to hold them to account.

And so if we, as a group, wanting to fight for the restoration and future of the NHS, are to successfully challenge what politicians are doing, we will need to be clear in our demands, and strategic in our actions. The first thing to do is to be clear about why we are doing this in the first place. The NHS, 75 years old, is one of the institutions most valued by the people of the UK. It exists to support and improve the health of every single person, and it has had a positive impact on millions upon millions of people during its long history.

Even at its inception, there were many politicians and others who vehemently opposed its existence. And that opposition to the NHS has continued through the decades, ebbing and flowing depending on the political landscape of the time, but always there in the background. This is specifically why the reforms that have brought us to this point, to the collapse of the NHS, have been enacted quietly. Politicians have always understood that there would be an enormous backlash if they were open and honest about their intentions. It is only now, at the point of wholesale collapse, as patients are being failed and are dying needlessly in large numbers because of the system's inability to keep them safe, that we see honesty from the politicians.

Because this is what we're seeing now, finally. Honesty from Rishi Sunak and Sajid Javid (and no doubt others in the near future), explaining that they think the NHS should introduce patient charges. They wouldn't have got away with saying that 10 years ago. They think they'll get away with it now because of the terrible state of the service. People are desperate, and some politicians think they are desperate enough to try anything in the hope of improving the situation.

But through its long tenure, its 75-year history of ups and downs, the public has been consistent about the fact that it values the service and wants it to continue. I think the government has underestimated the general public's current strength of feeling; its anger about the state of our society, the dismantling of the welfare state, the worsening quality of life for so many people, and the broader political landscape that has been marred by disgraced politicians, tax scandals, the breaking of rules and a failure to support the population properly. The public is very, very unhappy about what is going on.

Politicians have chosen to show their cards regarding the NHS, the Conservative Party in speaking about charging patients, and the Labour Party in talking about their hopes to utilise the private sector in supporting the NHS to recover. From what I'm seeing online, the thousands of people I'm speaking to, this isn't what the public wants. There is the sense that energy is building now, building to push back en masse.

The NHS was set up as a bold, progressive project, aiming to create equal healthcare that is comprehensive and free at the point of use. These were always ambitious goals, and they were always going to involve a constant reimagining of what the public needed. But these goals have never seemed more ambitious than right now, when staff in many places are unable to provide patients even with basic care. The long-term aim must be to fully attain these goals, to create a situation in which the three core principles are central to decision-making, and the NHS is able to take greater strides towards breaking down structural barriers within our society and offering everyone the care they need.

Right now, we must demand that the work begins to rebuild our NHS, shore it up, and strengthen both the infrastructure and the NHS workforce immediately, both to safeguard lives in the short term and to build sustainability within the public service. The first, and most obvious thing we could be doing to improve things would be to support staff. NHS staff are the backbone of the service, they keep it running, yet they are being wholly unsupported, which is causing more and more of them to leave.

We need the opposite to happen; we need staff to return. Those who have left the NHS workforce (either to work in the private sector, or move abroad, or retire) need to be attracted back. And those who are currently working within the NHS require support.

Staffing of the NHS is one of our biggest challenges. NHS staff have not been well supported in recent years, both during the height of the pandemic, when so many frontline workers endured an enormous burden of trauma without sufficient protection, and in their day-to-day work. When I speak to staff online, I hear continually about low morale and exhaustion that is affecting staff across the service. This is obviously in part to do with the treatment that individuals are receiving; they're not being paid properly for their skills, and are facing ever more pressure as the service buckles under the increasing waiting lists. But there's also a deep discomfort from staff in doing a job where they are no longer able to provide the type of care to their patients that makes them feel proud and satisfied in doing their work. Most healthcare professionals go into this line of work because, despite the challenges, it is a deeply rewarding experience to care for people and to help them live healthier lives. As the funding has been cut and the service has become progressively fragmented, their ability to care for people properly has diminished. This is a source of significant moral injury for a lot of staff members.

Staff across the board need to be given a substantial and immediate pay rise, both to restore the real-terms pay cuts that have been made over the past 13 years, and to redress the imbalance between healthcare worker wages paid in the UK, and those paid in other countries that are comparable from an economic standpoint. Hospital consultants in Ireland are now paid around three times as much as NHS consultant doctors, and this situation plays out in many other countries too. Working conditions for healthcare workers abroad are better in other ways too. Lower numbers of hours. More time to rest. Support with training budgets, allowing the work-force to keep up to date with the latest knowledge easily. All of these things support a workforce, and the NHS has fallen behind other countries on them for many years now.

It's not all about money. Staff have endured so much, and continue to do so, working in a system under huge pressure, before the pandemic, through the pandemic, and beyond. There are some fantastic projects and charities that support NHS workers with mental health support, but these need to be expanded and made more accessible to any staff member who needs support. Even when things are 'normal', working in healthcare is intense. There are sights you see and things you experience that become normalised, even though they aren't normal at all; they can be traumatic and they stay with healthcare workers. We need to do a much better job of caring for our workforce. Because, after all, if we're not caring for the staff, how can we expect them to be able to care well for their patients?

I speak to NHS staff every day about their experiences working within the NHS. And when they talk to me about what's really getting them down, keeping them awake at night through worry, it's issues relating to their patients and their colleagues. There is an incredible culture within the NHS; a culture of teamwork and responsibility, with countless people dedicated to doing the best they can for patients. But this culture has been taken advantage of in recent years. Staff have been expected to give more and more of themselves simply to keep the service going. It's not safe and it's not sustainable. Healthcare workers are trained to work well under pressure, and periods of heightened activity are expected by the staff. But the pressures simply never let up now.

I speak to a lot of frontline doctors about what is happening in both their professional and their personal lives. And as I write this I have had two emails in the past 24 hours from different doctors working in different specialities, both telling me that the stress and mental exhaustion associated with their jobs have led to depression and suicidal ideation in the past six months, and that if it wasn't for support (which they were forced to pay for privately), they think they would have taken their own lives. It requires a lot for anyone to admit that to another person, and because the NHS values qualities of 'resilience' and 'strength' and simply putting up with things, it can be very difficult to acknowledge how bad things have got. I have heard from both of these doctors because, now that they are recovering, they are determined to speak up and ensure that other doctors are not placed in the same position as them.

It is enormously brave of them to do this. I am so glad that both are in recovery now, but others aren't. We have a mental health crisis among healthcare professionals on our hands. There has been a slew of articles written recently about the mental health crisis among NHS staff, and what can be done about it. We must thank and celebrate the projects that already exist to support healthcare workers, including the Practitioner Health Programme,[9] and Doctors in Distress.[10] But much more needs to be done. We have to do a much better job of caring for our workforce. The Laura Hyde Foundation, which is an organisation that was set up in memory of a Royal Navy nurse, 'saw a 550% rise in demand for clinical mental health support from medical staff in 2020. The charity ... said that two healthcare workers die by suicide every week on average, while a doctor takes their own life once every three weeks.'[11]

And on top of treating the current workforce well, to encourage retention of staff, we need to train more staff fast. Recent years have seen a large exodus of staff members from the NHS workforce; and so it is urgent now to attract and recruit more people into the professions. The government has recently limited the number of places at medical school; this is completely the wrong policy. We should, instead, be training more healthcare professionals, and as part of this scheme the government should be widening the access of students entering the profession. We need a more diverse group of people entering healthcare professions, and we need to do far more to help students from disadvantaged backgrounds to become doctors, nurses and to enter the other allied health professions too.

And so our first priority, our immediate priority, is the staff; supporting the current workforce, and attracting new members of staff to strengthen the NHS at this time of crisis. Crucially, in all of this, the government needs to stop treating staff as commodities, taking every last ounce of energy from them, failing to show appreciation and expecting them to sacrifice more and more for less and less. We need to value staff, who are a group of highly trained professionals that we are so lucky to have. Their skills and expertise are incredibly valuable, and they are workers. They deserve to be valued and paid properly, just like all workers.

Beyond supporting and building the NHS workforce, there are a number of other areas in which immediate action could and should be taken to strengthen the NHS in the immediate future. The first is to urgently address the lack of capital investment in the service, which is why many of the NHS's buildings are in such bad shape.

No public healthcare system should be operating with crumbling buildings, leaking roofs and other problems, some of which have been deemed to carry a significant risk to staff and patients alike. The maintenance bill for unmet repairs in the NHS in England was £9 billion in June 2022[12] and this figure has been growing fast. The government has somehow managed to disregard the problems and failed to take responsibility. This needs to be addressed as a matter of urgency.

A flash poll of health leaders run by the NHS Confederation in June 2022 showed the scale of the current problems. The organisation explained at the time: 'NHS leaders warn of ageing buildings, run-down estate and outdated computer systems which are risking patient safety.' A provider Trust Chair had observed: 'The standard of much of our office accommodation and IT is miles behind the rest of the economy, we have constant problems with blocked toilets and our changing rooms and rest areas for staff are cramped and lack privacy. We are also not building up our capacity to deal with waiting lists, and the conditions for patients in some wards and clinics are not fit for purpose.'[13] The problems are happening all over. If we want the NHS to be able to function safely, the government needs to start investing in these basic things fast. These have been neglected for far too long, and the situation is contributing to patient safety problems now.

Alongside the maintenance upkeep, NHS PFI debt needs to be urgently paid off. Because of the PFI contracts that were entered into many years ago, some

NHS Trusts are in staggering amounts of debt, and it is affecting their financial stability. As the *Guardian* reported in October 2022: 'Hospital groups spent £2.3bn on legacy PFI projects in 2020–21, of which just under £1bn went on costs for essential services such as cleaning and maintenance. A third of the remaining PFI spend – £457m – went purely on paying off interest charges.'[14] The situation is perfectly summed up by David Rowland from the Centre for Health and the Public Interest, who stated in the piece:

> For those trusts with a PFI hospital, the high costs of these schemes will continue to be a major drain on their budgets. This is at a time when they are making planned cuts of £12bn a year and expect to have to meet an additional £6bn of costs next year due to inflation.
>
> Despite the pressure on NHS Trusts to make cuts, under the 25-year-long contract, PFI companies and their shareholders have been given a watertight guarantee that they will receive payments and a return on their investment. In short, expenditure on staff, equipment and other capital projects can be cut by a Trust, but not their PFI payments.
>
> In addition, under the PFI contracts the NHS Trusts, not the private companies, bear the risk of high inflation – which means that the payments to PFI companies may increase substantially as the retail price index rises. The rise in inflation

will consequently not dent substantially, if at all,
the profits of PFI companies.[15]

The situation is appalling. Some of the PFI contracts run
almost to 2050, and despite repeated calls from
campaigners in recent years to end the schemes and pay
off the money, the government has ignored this. We are
in a situation that is financially scuppering some NHS
Trusts, who are forced to squeeze their spending in other
areas in order to pay the PFI bills every year. This money
could be put to better use; for example, improving things
for patients.

As explained by the *New Statesman*, 'Government
figures from 2018 show the value of the initial PFI
investments in the NHS was just £12.8bn, but the
Department for Health and Social Care will have spent
a total £80.7bn once they are all paid off'[16] (this figure
includes services such as facilities management supplied
by the PFI providers).The government needs to find a
way to pay off this PFI debt, fast.

These issues – strengthening the staff workforce,
doing the basic repairs and upkeep, and paying off the
PFI debt – are the immediate priorities, and could be
achieved in the short term through immediate investment from the government. Until they are done, it is
difficult to focus on the bigger picture. The day-to-
day running of the service needs to be improved before
any broader conversations about it can properly take
place.

Once those three things have been achieved, we need
to return to NHS principles and think bigger. The NHS

was set up as an ambitious project; a project that was intended to keep our population healthy, and provide equal, comprehensive provision of healthcare across the country. The current state of the system, with thousands of services run by private providers, some of which may be leading to patient safety failings, as well as creating the churn and disruption of short-term contracts, are not serving the public. They create patchy service delivery across the country, they interfere with long-term caring relationships between staff and patients, and they do not create sustainability within our public healthcare system.

A conversation that seems to be missed when people talk about the fragmentation of our health service is the loss, amid this outsourcing, of the built knowledge and experience within the service itself. Many NHS staff aim to work within the service for many years, or their entire career. And when you are working within the service, these people, the services they run, the processes they develop, the knowledge they bring to their work of the local population and their needs, is unbelievably rich. The value of this cannot be underestimated. When a new provider comes in and wins a contract to run an NHS service, often they disrupt this built knowledge and the careful processes that have been developed over time by the NHS staff who understand their patient populations. It is a metric that goes unmeasured, but the loss is profound.

And when the ethos is competition; when providers are intent on pushing competitors out of the way and winning these NHS contracts, something else is lost too. The NHS was a service built on collaboration and shared learning. Outsourcing destroys this ethos. If a provider comes in and starts to build up its own processes, its own built knowledge of a population, but then doesn't renew its contract, loses the contract to a competitor, or decides to extricate itself from one because it is not profitable for the company to continue, this built knowledge is lost. Our healthcare system should be retaining the built knowledge of healthcare professionals working with their population. We should not be allowing this information to be lost, only to be re-learned by the next outsourced provider, or the one after that. It is a waste, and it impacts on how well patients are understood and ultimately the care they will receive from their local services.

If we want the NHS to thrive for another 75 years, and to achieve the aims it set out to fulfil, we need to eliminate outsourcing from the NHS. It must be stopped and reversed. Often when I am speaking about this online, people point out that achieving this will take a lot of effort, work and time. First, I think they underestimate the current effort that is being expended in tendering contracts for these outsourced providers. The sheer administration involved in the tendering of NHS contracts creates a huge amount of work across the country; work that could be done away with if we invested in the idea that we want our public healthcare system to be publicly funded and run. And second, I don't think we should be intimidated by an ambitious plan to return the NHS to the structure and shape that was intended at its inception. It has taken four long decades for politicians to implement the many changes that have brought us to where we are. It might take a while and a lot of effort to get back to the functioning we require; but the long-term benefits for the service and patients will be enormous, and it is the best way to ensure the NHS's viability, sustainability and progress for the decades to come.

There are so many challenges facing our society and, by the same merit, facing the NHS, and we will be best placed to tackle these once the service has been brought back into full public ownership. Perhaps the most obvious of these is technology. As described above, due to a lack of capital investment over many years, the NHS has fallen far behind on its tech investment. There is a huge disconnect at present between the level of technology that our society has developed, and what staff are working with in the NHS. In terms of patient healthcare, the service has always been at the cutting edge of available science and medicine, which is a source of great pride for many people.

But in terms of IT structures, essential to help services to run efficiently and to aid communication between healthcare teams, we are lagging far behind. In the early 2000s, the Labour Party created a 'National Programme for IT', which was intended to 'revolutionise the way the health service worked'. But the project turned into utter chaos and a waste of taxpayer money to the tune of £10bn.[17] It was a disaster involving changing requirements, delays and technical challenges. The project ran years behind time and was eventually abandoned. And since then, politicians seem to have lost their ambitions regarding technology within the NHS.

When politicians in recent years have spoken positively about the use of technology and AI, it has seemingly attracted enthusiasm mostly as a way of instilling yet more privatisation into the service. Matt Hancock during his tenure as Health Secretary was very keen to emphasise his enthusiasm for new technology, most notably in his promotion of Babylon (the private healthcare company mentioned earlier that won NHS contracts to deliver an online app for GP appointments called 'GP at hand'). If we want to fight for an NHS that will not just survive, but thrive in years to come, we need to push politicians to invest in the technology that the NHS owns, not simply encourage more external providers to take on NHS contracts. Because, of course, when an external company runs an NHS service, they own the technology and the developments that they make. It means that if they end their contracts with the NHS (as Babylon has done on several occasions[18]) the knowledge from the project does not remain in the NHS; it is lost. We need to be investing heavily in technology that is developed and owned by the NHS, to ensure that the public service benefits from it in the long term.

Technology that is owned by one private company or another is also limited in terms of information sharing across the NHS. In 2022, despite the wealth of technology that we have in our society, there are still huge limitations whereby clinicians in one part of the country struggle to readily access information about NHS patients in a different part. There isn't a single, joined-up IT system. Technology has the power to improve connectivity and improve people's health. It is important therefore that the NHS receives the investment to improve the technology within the service.

And in thinking about key structures within the NHS that would need enormous, much-needed investment, another obvious area is the 'NHS estate'. The buildings that make up NHS facilities are a hodgepodge of buildings of differing ages, some of which are older than the NHS itself and which were bought at the NHS's inception. Healthcare needs have changed enormously over the past 75 years. Scanning technology has changed enormously. Operating theatres have changed. Intensive care units did not used to exist. The set-up of wards has changed, and as medical advances have occurred over the decades, there has been the need for more and more departments incorporating new and differing equipment. When new buildings have been designed, planners and architects have tried at various junctures to design new structures in versatile ways. But many of the buildings are now poorly organised, and this has led to crowding, uncomfortable working environments, and inefficiencies in delivering good care.

Many of the buildings are also poorly ventilated, or draughty, or overheated. There is a running joke among NHS staff that there are two temperatures within NHS buildings; roasting (to the point that staff are often forced to open the windows to reduce the temperature because it gets so uncomfortable) or freezing. This is energy-inefficient and uncomfortable for the huge number of people, both staff and patients, who operate within the buildings. It's also irresponsible in 2023; important questions are starting to be asked about the impact of the NHS on the climate emergency, and the costly waste of energy within the service. Amid a cost-of-living crisis so extreme that many local areas are setting up 'warm banks' and places where people can go to escape their freezing homes, the management of energy within the NHS is becoming more and more pertinent.

Staff are starting to raise concerns about the situation. During the heatwave of 2022, I heard from a number who were forced into working in inhumane conditions, with temperatures in their offices above 30°C. This was hard enough for the staff, because temperatures like this do not make it easy for people to concentrate. But it was even worse for the patients, many of whom of course would already have been feeling unwell. We were sent various examples of air-conditioning units breaking, and in one A&E department staff started fainting from the heat.

Politicians are going to have to start making long-term planning decisions to tackle these significant problems within the NHS's structure and functioning. It is absolutely imperative if we want the service to continue in the decades to come.

The NHS has other huge challenges to face up to. Millions of patients are facing barriers in accessing NHS treatment at present. The situation is shocking for so many. But the barriers faced will not be equal. We are living in a society with significant structural barriers affecting many groups of people. Conversations about inequity of care and structural barriers need to become much more prominent. If we are to succeed in rebuilding this public healthcare system and ensuring that it is fit for the next 75 years, these issues are absolutely central. There needs to be a reconsideration of the leadership within the NHS; who is making the decisions, on behalf of which patients. Active efforts need to be made to hear from patient groups that are insufficiently heard, and there needs to be much more done to ensure that leadership roles are held by a diverse group of individuals, matching the diversity of our population. It is the only way we can hope to provide good care to our communities.

We have ended up where we are, with a dysfunctional and poorly managed service, heavily infiltrated with privatisation, because decisions from one government that do not serve the public are stacked onto the decisions of previous governments, which also did not serve us. The reforms have been enacted gradually, in a stepwise manner, to bring us to where we are today. The NHS has been steered down a different path; and our public healthcare project is now very far off course. But the changes we require are clear.

It is undeniable that these necessary changes will be enormously costly. Investing in hospital buildings, paying off PFI debt, paying staff properly, building the technology we need, tackling the sustainability within the service, ending out-sourcing and buying up the parts of the NHS that have already been sold off will be difficult, and expensive, and will require some new legislation to be written. And beyond this, the investment needed to tackle structural barriers and rebuild a system whereby the full diversity of our society is reflected in NHS leadership and direction would be a huge investment.

The money involved, the staggering sums, are difficult to estimate. The NHS still owes around £50 billion simply in PFI debts, and all of the above goals would be hugely expensive to enact, in part because so much has been neglected for so long. When ideas such as these are proposed by campaigners, the question of costs commonly comes up, and many conclude that such bold plans have no hope of being enacted because we simply do not have the money as a country to pay for them.

I am not an economist, and I am not going to attempt to estimate the sums required to bring the NHS back to the level of functioning required. But to my mind, this is not a question of costs, it is one of priority. Polling of the public has consistently shown that it supports the continuation of the NHS. The health service also has a clear constitution that it is currently failing to adhere to; we do not at present have a public healthcare system that is delivering comprehensive care to all. So the government has two options (because it has no mandate to continue along a trajectory that is causing the NHS to fail on its own principles). It must either accept that its plans are not working and embrace bold ideas for radical, transformative change, or it must hold a referendum regarding the abolition of the NHS constitution (which it is no longer adhering to).

It is quite clear to my mind what the outcome of that referendum would be. The British public cares deeply about the NHS and I highly doubt it would agree with getting rid of its constitution. So where does that leave us? It leaves us in the position of needing to find the money to rebuild the NHS. And I do not believe this to be the hopeless situation that it is often framed to be. It is true that our public finances are in dire straits. But in the years following the Second World War, when the NHS was first started, the country was facing even bigger, more complex challenges. And the will of the populace won out. That traumatised post-war landscape, ravaged by war and with enormous financial challenges, is the landscape in which the NHS was built. It can be rebuilt again. Taxes for wealthy people may need to be raised. Other, less important projects may have to be delayed, or reined in, to enable the NHS investment required. But what is more important to our society than the health of our nation and the well-being of every person? Nothing, to my mind. After all, the benefits of a healthy society span far, far beyond the individual benefits of any person's lack of illness. A healthy population can lead to a larger labour force, greater productivity and a healthier economy.

Despite what the government clearly should be doing, it is highly unlikely it will choose to take this course of action, so it will be up to all of us who care about the NHS to push them into action. And our campaign will need to be bold; communicating to as many people as possible what our demands are and why it is important. A proactive campaign, speaking in hopeful terms about what we want, and the benefits it will create for everyone, will be the most effective course of action. We need energy, enthusiasm and confidence. I have learned over my years of campaigning that while people will often take an immediate action (like signing a petition) in the short term out of fear or anger, the campaigns that yield the most powerful long-term impacts are those that have a sense of hope; where people are working towards a future that they want to be a part of. Those are the campaigns that really fly, that capture the imagination of many people and create real and lasting change.

Those who have taken action to speak up about the NHS generally do so for a reason. Often there's a memory of something that has stuck with them, and it resonated sufficiently to cause their mindset to shift. For some people it might have been a personal encounter within the NHS, a time when they realised the value of the service, or its failings. For others, it could be a change that has happened locally; for example, the closure of a GP surgery or the threatened closure of their hospital.

My mindset shifted during one night shift when I was working as a junior psychiatry doctor. On our night shifts we carried out assessments for new patients and assessed emergencies in a mental health hospital, as well as assessing patients in the A&E department and wards of a busy London teaching hospital that was about half a mile up the road. There's something about night shifts that feels distinctly different to day shifts in a hospital. It's unnatural to be awake at 3am, and I always found my patient encounters overnight to be starker somehow. And this was particularly true when working in the emergency department. Being in an A&E department is an uncomfortable experience at any time of day for patients, but to be there in the middle of the night talking to a doctor is especially hard. No one wants to be doing that.

I was called at about 3am to see a new patient in the A&E department. It was cold that night, and I was in our office across the road at the time. I remember crossing the road to A&E to see my next patient. He was a homeless man who had attended the A&E department because he was feeling suicidal. Psychiatry assessments are quite lengthy, and I spent about an hour speaking to him to assess how serious his symptoms were. He felt terrible, and he was having a very hard time that was made even more difficult because he had nowhere to stay and was sleeping rough. However, he didn't have an active plan to harm himself. We were incredibly short of hospital beds and so the bar had been incrementally raised higher and higher in terms of how unwell a patient would need to be to be granted a hospital admission. I saw a lot of patients who would have benefited from a hospital admission, and so did all of my colleagues. But we simply didn't have the resources to provide this.

And so I discussed the situation with my senior doctor colleague, and I discharged this man, telling him that our community team would be in touch to arrange an appointment. But as I watched this man walk out of the emergency department, I felt deeply ashamed. I had spent over an hour speaking to him about his problems and assessing him. And he wasn't well; he just wasn't sufficiently unwell to warrant an admission that night, and I had nothing else to offer him. It felt deeply wrong that we hadn't offered him more help, and deeply uncaring. We simply didn't have enough care to give. I think about this patient frequently. That interaction caused something to shift for me. My mindset changed and never went back. And it did so for one very simple reason; we were not providing good care.

I'm not alone in having an experience like this. When I speak to people who in various ways are speaking up about the NHS and the actions of politicians, they inevitably have a moment they can identify when something shifted in their mindset too. Maybe it was when their mum needed care and the ambulance didn't come. Or perhaps it did come, and this care made a deep impression upon them, and they don't want anyone else in a similar position to be denied this level of care. I've never met anyone whose mindset changed because they read a particular headline or saw a graph showing how things in the NHS are worsening. Graphs and numbers are important, but in my experience people only start getting worried about the graphs and the numbers once they're already worried about patient care, or a lack of it.

I've been campaigning long enough to know that a lot of people will make all kinds of disparaging noises if you start to talk about care. They will attempt to undermine the notion that it matters. There are countless people – MPs, journalists and others – who believe there is some better measure of healthcare outcomes, and that talking about care somehow misses the point, and focuses on something gauzy and unimportant. But I absolutely disagree with that. Some patients receive adequate, safe treatment that in terms of health outcome could be judged as sufficient, but that didn't feel particularly caring to them. But if we want to be running an excellent healthcare system – one where people feel they have the time to explain things and feel heard, and staff have the space to listen, and patients have access to all of the allied healthcare professionals to provide excellent treatment and a good recovery – that system will feel caring.

So, if we are going to push back against everything the politicians are doing, we need to bring the conversation back to care. Care is the most basic and most important element of our healthcare system. Patients and staff need to come together now; we are not in opposition. Everyone would be much happier if the service was being run excellently and there was enough care to go around. If we are going to fight, then, for the NHS, we need to ask a lot of people one very basic question – staff and patients: 'Do you think the NHS is caring for people properly?' Anyone who says 'no' is someone who will potentially take action to change things.

Most people aren't sure of all the facts, but feel let down. And those people, despite some of them having absorbed unhelpful rhetoric from the media or from politicians, are seeking answers. The only way we are going to win this is if we can break down the barriers, start conversations, and talk to the many people who feel let down and have had their anger diverted away from the government. Every single member of the public deserves compassion right now, because every single person has been failed.

The only thing that will stop the politicians' betrayal of the NHS is us. You and me and everyone who cares about the service and its future. We are living through extraordinary times, a time of political discord and chaos, of divisions and difficulties, where so many people don't have enough and have been let down in countless ways by a government that tries to get away with as much as it can without scrutiny, without transparency, without accountability to the people it serves. But extraordinary times give rise to extraordinary ideas.

The NHS was an extraordinary idea that came into being because a huge number of people believed that our society should be providing good care for every single person in their hour of need. That idea was transformative at the time, and that same idea has the power to improve lives and the health of our entire population today. We can rebuild the NHS, ending the private outsourcing, supporting the staff, fixing the problems, listening and learning and reimagining what our society needs from our public healthcare system.

As William Beveridge said in his report in 1942, the report that helped to give rise to the NHS in the first place: 'A revolutionary moment in the world's history is a time for revolutions, not for patching.'[19] From this global pandemic, we face another revolutionary moment. It's not a time for more concessions, small changes, or compromises. It's time for the bold, transformative ideas that will help us to rebuild the NHS to thrive for the next 75 years. It's time to fight for the NHS.

ACKNOWLEDGEMENTS

Thank you so much to my wonderful editor Anna Mrowiec, all the team at HarperCollins for helping this book to become a reality, and to Nick Fawcett, who copy-edited the manuscript. Thank you to the EveryDoctor team, past and present, to the TPM team, and especially to my fellow directors Dr Georgina Wood and Dr Megan Smith. Thank you to every single person who is fighting for the future of the NHS. And thank you to the N.N.C. – every day, now and forever. You fill my days with laughter and light.

FURTHER READING

There are many fantastic resources about the NHS and NHS privatisation, and many wonderful campaigning organisations doing incredible work. I've listed several key resources here if you're interested in learning more.

1. Youssef El-Gingihy's book *How to Dismantle the NHS in 10 Easy Steps*
2. John Pilger's documentary *The Dirty War on the NHS*
3. Dr Bob Gill's documentary *The Great NHS Heist*
4. The 'Your NHS Needs You' campaign – www.yournhsneedsyou.com
5. EveryDoctor's map of privatisation and outsourcing – www.everydoctor.org.uk

If you'd like to follow me for updates, I'm @JujuliaGrace on Twitter. I write a personal newsletter on Substack. You can subscribe by going to jujuliagrace.substack.com.

REFERENCES

INTRODUCTION

1. https://www.theguardian.com/world/2020/may/31/how-a
-decade-of-privatisation-and-cuts-exposed-england-to-coronavirus £81
billion was to be cut over the next five years

2. https://www.newstatesman.com/business/economics/2012/12
/osborne-cutting-nhs-not-deficit

3. https://www.theguardian.com/world/2020/may/31/how-a
-decade-of-privatisation-and-cuts-exposed-england-to-coronavirus

4. https://www.kingsfund.org.uk/publications/articles/government
-pledge-seven-day-services

5. https://www.theguardian.com/society/2016/aug/23/jeremy-hunt
-weekend-nhs-death-claims-unhelpful-say-civil-servants

6. https://www.indy100.com/celebrities/junior-doctors-are-posting
-pictures-to-disprove-the-sun-s-moet-medics-story-7288226

7. https://www.youtube.com/watch?v=MFl5yB6_9OI

8. https://www.independent.co.uk/news/uk/politics/junior-doctors
-outraged-over-new-contract-that-discriminates-against-single-women
-a6963356.html

9. https://www.theguardian.com/society/2016/feb/11/jeremy-hunt
-to-impose-contract-on-junior-doctors

10. https://www.theguardian.com/society/2020/mar/31/nhs-staff-gagged-over-coronavirus-protective-equipment-shortages; https://www.theguardian.com/society/2020/mar/16/not-fit-for-purpose-uk-medics-condemn-covid-19-protection

11. https://www.ons.gov.uk/peoplepopulationandcommunity/births deathsandmarriages/deaths/adhocs/14379deathsinvolvingcorona viruscovid19amonghealthandsocialcareworkersthoseaged20to 64yearsenglandandwalesdeathsregistered9march2020to28 february2022; https://www.amnesty.org.uk/press-releases/uk-among-highest-covid-19-health-worker-deaths-world; https://www.theguardian.com/world/2020/apr/20/at-least-100-uk-health-workers-have-died-from-coronavirus-figures-show

12. https://smk.org.uk/awards_nominations/protectnhsworkers/

13. https://www.bbc.com/news/uk-england-nottinghamshire-52025950

CHAPTER 1

1. https://www.telegraph.co.uk/columnists/2022/06/09/lauded-nhs-pandemic-just-naive/

2. https://www.theguardian.com/politics/2023/jan/20/sajid-javid-calls-for-patients-to-pay-for-gp-and-ae-visits

3. https://www.cnbc.com/2019/02/11/this-is-the-real-reason-most-americans-file-for-bankruptcy.html

4. https://www.ipsos.com/en-uk/what-makes-us-proud-be-british

5. https://www.ons.gov.uk/peoplepopulationandcommunity/births deathsandmarriages/lifeexpectancies/bulletins/nationallifetablesunited kingdom/2018to2020

6. https://www.bbc.com/news/health-42572110

7. https://www.bbc.com/news/health-44560590

8. https://www.parliament.uk/about/living-heritage/transforming society/livinglearning/coll-9-health1/coll-9-health/

REFERENCES

9. https://www.parliament.uk/about/living-heritage/transforming society/private-lives/yourcountry/collections/collections-second -world-war/parliamentarians-and-people/clement-attlee/

10. https://navigator.health.org.uk/theme/national-insurance-act -1911

11. https://www.instituteforgovernment.org.uk/explainer/devolution -and-nhs

12. https://www.theguardian.com/society/2016/apr/01/female -doctors-new-contract-medical-royal-colleges

13. https://www.everydoctor.org.uk/nhs-privatisation-map

14. https://fullfact.org/health/what-nhs-paying-private-finance -initiatives/; https://www.theguardian.com/politics/2019/sep/12 /nhs-hospital-trusts-to-pay-out-further-55bn-under-pfi-scheme

15. https://www.theguardian.com/commentisfree/2021/oct/15/tory -austerity-deaths-cut-human-cost-cruel-policy

16. https://www.theguardian.com/society/2021/oct/14/austerity-in -england-linked-to-more-than-50000-extra-deaths-in-five-years

17. https://www.theguardian.com/society/2022/may/31/loss -of-25000-nhs-beds-caused-serious-patient-safety-crisis-finds-report

18. https://nursingnotes.co.uk/news/years-of-austerity-sees-nhs-workers -up-to-32-worse-off-than-ten-years-ago-new-data-reveals

19. https://www.theguardian.com/society/2016/jul/21/nhs-bursaries -for-student-nurses-will-end-in-2017-government-confirms

20. https://news.sky.com/story/first-victory-in-campaign-to-restore -student-nurse-grants-11889437

21. https://www.theguardian.com/society/2022/jun/14/rundown -nhs-hospitals-have-become-a-danger-to-patients-warn-health-chiefs

22. https://www.theguardian.com/society/2017/jan/06/nhs-faces -humanitarian-crisis-rising-demand-british-red-cross

23. https://www.nuffieldtrust.org.uk/resource/how-much-is-covid-19 -to-blame-for-growing-nhs-waiting-times

24. https://www.theguardian.com/society/2020/apr/26/more-than -two-million-operations-cancelled-as-nhs-fights-covid-19

25. https://www.england.nhs.uk/2021/02/nhs-expands-mental-health-support-for-staff-after-toughest-year-in-health-service-history/

26. https://www.everydoctor.org.uk/blog/everydoctors-2021-recap

27. https://www.theguardian.com/world/2020/dec/04/gps-in-england-told-to-prepare-vaccination-sites-for-mid-december

28. https://www.england.nhs.uk/2021/01/nhs-organisations-instructed-to-rapidly-vaccinate-staff/, https://www.everydoctor.org.uk/blog/everydoctors-2021-recap

29. https://www.nuffieldtrust.org.uk/resource/how-much-is-covid-19-to-blame-for-growing-nhs-waiting-times

30. https://news.sky.com/story/nhs-waiting-list-hits-record-high-of-7-2-million-people-as-almost-third-of-patients-wait-four-hours-in-a-e-12763943

31. https://news.sky.com/story/nhs-more-than-1-000-people-waiting-longer-than-12-hours-in-a-e-every-day-figures-reveal-12633551

32. https://www.health.org.uk/publications/long-reads/why-have-ambulance-waiting-times-been-getting-worse

33. https://www.theguardian.com/society/2023/jan/12/ae-patients-in-england-waiting-over-12-hours-top-50000-for-first-time

34. https://www.instituteforgovernment.org.uk/article/comment/boris-johnson-must-now-deliver-his-promised-plan-fix-social-care, https://commonslibrary.parliament.uk/research-briefings/cbp-8001/

35. https://www.theguardian.com/society/2022/nov/13/hospital-beds-england-occupied-patients-fit-discharge

36. https://www.kingsfund.org.uk/publications/what-does-public-think-about-nhs

CHAPTER 2

1. https://www.thetimes.co.uk/article/state-cant-fix-all-your-problems-says-rishi-sunak-6vlw6q3bw

REFERENCES

2. https://www.bbc.com/news/uk-63429244

3. https://www.itv.com/news/tyne-tees/2022-07-21/rishi-sunak-treats-journalists-to-twix-sprite-and-suncream-for-the-road

4. https://www.theguardian.com/commentisfree/2022/oct/05/liz-truss-tory-party-conference-speech-thatcherism; https://www.newstatesman.com/quickfire/2022/10/rishi-sunak-thatcherite-prime-minister-since-thatcher

5. https://www.independent.co.uk/news/health/nhs-accident-emergency-deaths-strikes-nurses-b2254523.html

6. https://www.independent.co.uk/news/uk/politics/jeremy-hunt-privatise-nhs-tories-privatising-private-insurance-market-replacement-direct-democracy-a6865306.html

7. https://www.theguardian.com/society/2019/may/12/nhs-pensions-trap-plan-to-halt-exodus-angry-doctors-contribtutions

8. https://www.hsj.co.uk/comment/the-bedpan-safe-in-the-iron-ladys-hands/7026198.article

9. https://www.theguardian.com/society/2022/nov/27/no-10-hiring-of-private-healthcare-lobbyist-prompts-privatisation-concern

10. https://www.opendemocracy.net/en/elective-recovery-taskforce-private-healthcare-nhs/

11. https://news.sky.com/story/hancock-committed-minor-breach-of-ministerial-code-when-covid-contract-awarded-to-sisters-company-12319324

12. https://www.theguardian.com/politics/2018/nov/30/matt-hancock-accused-of-breaching-code-over-gp-app-endorsement

13. https://www.theguardian.com/politics/2021/jun/22/shareholders-of-firm-backed-by-matt-hancock-have-donated-to-the-tories

14. https://www.mirror.co.uk/news/politics/tories-raking-money-private-health-29017569

15. https://www.standard.co.uk/news/uk/health-secretary-matt-hancock-reveals-deeply-personal-connection-to-the-nhs-a3892626.html

16. https://www.theguardian.com/healthcare-network/views-from
-the-nhs-frontline/2017/nov/16/seeing-gp-smartphone-sounds
-wonderful-its-not

17. https://www.theguardian.com/politics/2015/may/18/cameron
-seven-day-health-service-nhs-pledge-conservatives

18. https://www.nuffieldtrust.org.uk/news-item/the-brexit-referendum
-five-years-on-what-has-it-meant-for-the-nhs

19. https://www.theguardian.com/society/2022/apr/11/gp-numbers
-in-england-down-every-year-since-2015-pledge-to-raise-them

20. https://www.theguardian.com/society/2021/nov/02/no-10-set-to
-break-promise-of-6000-more-gps-in-england-sajid-javid-says

21. https://www.theguardian.com/society/2022/nov/14/sunak-omits
-target-of-6000-more-gps-from-brief-for-health-secretary

22. https://www.independent.co.uk/news/uk/politics/new
-hospitals-tory-manifesto-nhs-b2145857.html

23. https://www.bbc.com/news/59372348

24. Ibid.

25. Ibid.

26. https://www.theguardian.com/society/2023/feb/04/only
-10-of-boris-johnson-promised-40-new-hospitals-have-full-planning
-permission

27. https://www.dailymail.co.uk/news/article-8165745
/NHS-bowled-750-000-people-sign-volunteer-army-fight-coronavirus
.html

28. https://www.thesun.co.uk/news/13684742/volunteer-jabs-army
-pandemic-vaccine-sign-up-target-2/

29. https://www.independent.co.uk/news/uk/nhs-sajid-javid-nhs
-improvement-people-england-b2025826.html

30. https://www.theguardian.com/society/2022/sep/01/nhs-vacancies
-in-england-at-staggering-new-high-as-almost-10-of-posts-empty

31. https://nhscharitiestogether.co.uk

32. https://www.telegraph.co.uk/news/2022/03/18/department-health
-spend-almost-400m-management-consultants/

REFERENCES

33. https://blogs.lse.ac.uk/politicsandpolicy/using-management -consultancy-brings-inefficiency-to-the-nhs/

34. https://www.express.co.uk/news/uk/1415772/brexit-news-union -jack-hospitals-railways-police-stations

35. https://www.theguardian.com/society/2022/jun/11/nhs-needs -reform-not-more-money-to-deliver-sajid-javid-says

36. https://www.thetimes.co.uk/article/nhs-doesnt-need-cash-says -steve-barclay-999nrh5cz

37. https://www.reuters.com/world/uk/uks-opposition-labour-party -surges-33-point-lead-over-conservatives-yougov-poll-2022-09-29/

38. https://www.independent.co.uk/news/uk/politics/keir-starmer -nhs-pledge-privatisation-b2123849.html

39. https://labourlist.org/2022/07/some-private-provision-in -the-nhs-will-continue-under-labour-starmer-says/

40. https://www.spectator.co.uk/article/wes-streeting-keirs-not -superman-he-cant-do-it-all-by-himself/

41. https://www.theguardian.com/politics/2022/oct/28/hospital -patient-challenges-rishi-sunak-nurses-pay-catherine-poole

42. https://www.theguardian.com/politics/2022/dec/19/mother -steve-barclay-health-secretary-nhs-staff-waiting-lists-hospital

CHAPTER 3

1. https://www.specsavers.co.uk/eye-test/nhs-eye-test

2. https://www.everydoctor.org.uk/nhs-privatisation-map

3. https://www.legislation.gov.uk/ukpga/2022/31/contents/enacted

4. https://www.nationalhealthexecutive.com/articles/health -and-care-act-rubberstamped

5. https://www.england.nhs.uk/integratedcare/what-is-integrated -care/

6. https://www.gov.uk/government/publications/health-and-care -act-2022-combined-impact-assessments; https://committees.parliament

.uk/publications/6630/documents/72309/default/; https://www
.telegraph.co.uk/news/2021/02/11/matt-hancock-pledges-cut-nhs-bur
densome-bureaucracy-major-reforms/

7. https://www.nhsconfed.org/articles/were-told-nhs-protected
-cuts-alone-wont-save-it; https://www.theguardian.com/society/2021
/oct/14/austerity-in-england-linked-to-more-than-50000-extra
-deaths-in-five-years; https://www.gla.ac.uk/news/headline_885099
_en.html; https://www.kingsfund.org.uk/projects/impact-nhs-financial
-pressures-patient-care

8. https://www.bbc.co.uk/news/health-59865822

9. Ibid.

10. Ibid.

11. https://www.nhsconfed.org/news/nhs-leaders-facing-real-terms
-cut-funding-and-impossible-choices-over-which-areas-patient-care

12. https://www.theguardian.com/politics/2019/sep/12/nhs-hospital
-trusts-to-pay-out-further-55bn-under-pfi-scheme

13. https://www.newstatesman.com/spotlight/healthcare/2022/05
/pfi-repayments-are-costing-some-hospitals-twice-as-much-as-drugs

14. https://www.dailymail.co.uk/news/article-2077784/Labours
-botched-PFI-deals-sent-NHS-costs-soaring.html

15. https://www.theguardian.com/uk-news/2018/oct/29/hammond
-abolishes-pfi-contracts-for-new-infrastructure-projects

16. https://www.theguardian.com/society/2015/jan/09/circle-hospital
-private-firms-nhs-report-poor-care-hinchingbrooke

17. https://www.ft.com/content/502cf8fa-97d0-11e4-84d4-00144
feabdc0

18. https://www.standard.co.uk/futurelondon/health/matt-hancock-on
-ai-and-the-nhs-a3998006.html; https://www.theguardian.com/politics
/2021/jun/22/shareholders-of-firm-backed-by-matt-hancock-have-do
nated-to-the-tories

19. https://www.pulsetoday.co.uk/news/breaking-news/babylon-gp
-at-hand-to-quit-birmingham-affecting-5k-patients/; https://www

REFERENCES

.gpathand.nhs.uk; https://www.theguardian.com/society/2019/may/30/concerns-over-gp-at-hands-effect-on-local-primary-care-in-the-nhs

20. https://www.wired.co.uk/article/babylon-disrupted-uk-health-system-then-left

21. https://news.sky.com/story/matt-hancock-finishes-third-in-im-a-celebrity-get-me-out-of-here-12756886

22. https://www.hsj.co.uk/finance-and-efficiency/leaks-reveal-two-thirds-of-private-hospital-capacity-went-unused-by-nhs/7029000.article

23. https://www.mirror.co.uk/news/politics/private-hospitals-paid-millions-take-25900886

24. https://www.theguardian.com/business/2022/jan/13/private-health-firms-england-fight-omicron-surge-hospital-operators-services-nhs

25. https://www.bbc.com/news/health-44043959

26. https://blogs.lse.ac.uk/politicsandpolicy/nhs-spending-on-the-independent-sector/

27. https://www.theguardian.com/politics/2019/dec/13/bombastic-boris-johnson-wins-huge-majority-on-promise-to-get-brexit-done

28. https://metro.co.uk/2020/11/08/marcus-rashford-forces-another-government-u-turn-on-free-school-meals-13557307/; https://www.bbc.com/news/uk-53065806; https://www.theguardian.com/education/2020/nov/08/marcus-rashford-forces-boris-johnson-into-second-u-turn-on-child-food-poverty

29. https://www.newstatesman.com/business/2021/02/four-men-own-britain-s-news-media-problem-democracy

30. https://rcem.ac.uk/wp-content/uploads/2021/11/RCEM_Why_Emergency_Department_Crowding_Matters.pdf

31. https://www.theguardian.com/society/2021/nov/18/a-and-e-overcrowding-uk-deaths-year-doctors-treatment

32. https://www.nhsconfed.org

CRITICAL

33. https://www.theguardian.com/society/2019/nov/20/charities-call
-for-end-gagging-law-lobbying-act-run-up-elections

34. https://www.independent.co.uk/news/uk/politics/rnli-dominic
-raab-refugees-channel-migrants-b1893129.html

35. https://www.theguardian.com/commentisfree/2021/oct/14
/the-guardian-view-on-the-national-trust-battleground-for-a-culture
-war

36. https://www.everydoctor.org.uk

37. https://www.everydoctor.org.uk/blog/scrapnhsbill-setting
-mps-straight-part-1

38. https://apps.who.int/iris/bitstream/handle/10665/58
523/WHO_TFHE_TBN_95.1.pdf

39. https://www.theguardian.com/politics/2016/aug/23
/jeremy-corbyn-promise-renationalise-nhs-labour-private-end

40. https://www.independent.co.uk/news/uk/politics/keir-starmer
-nhs-pledge-privatisation-b2123849.html

41. https://www.bbc.com/news/uk-56400751

42. https://www.theguardian.com/media/2023/jan/11/national-security
-bill-may-have-chilling-effect-on-investigative-journalism-in-uk

43. https://www.yournhsneedsyou.com/renationalisation/

44. https://www.opendemocracy.net/en/ournhs/moment-of-honesty
-is-required-new-labour-began-dismantling-of-our-nhs/

45. https://www.theguardian.com/politics/2015/may/18
/cameron-seven-day-health-service-nhs-pledge-conservatives

46. https://www.theguardian.com/politics/2022/may/20/samantha
-jones-boris-johnson-downing-street-partygate

47. https://www.theguardian.com/society/2014/oct/23/simon
-stevens-nhs-chief-private-past-uk

48. https://www.england.nhs.uk/five-year-forward-view/

49. https://www.england.nhs.uk/publication/sustainability
-and-transformation-plan-footprints-march-2016/

50. https://www.theguardian.com/society/2022/nov/27/no-10-hiring
-of-private-healthcare-lobbyist-prompts-privatisation-concern

REFERENCES

CHAPTER 4

1. https://www.independent.co.uk/news/health/child-mental-health
-waiting-times-b1972830.html

2. https://www.bbc.com/news/education-48658151

3. https://www.itv.com/news/2016-01-11/david-cameron-to-promise
-1bn-mental-health-revolution

4. https://www.independent.co.uk/news/uk/politics/mental
-health-treatment-matt-hancock-conservative-government-awareness
-a8576796.html

5. https://www.aomrc.org.uk/wp-content/uploads/2022/09/Fixing
_the_NHS_210922.pdf

6. https://www.theguardian.com/world/2020/may/07/what-was
-exercise-cygnus-and-what-did-it-find

7. https://nursingnotes.co.uk/news/over-850-health-and-social-care
-workers-have-now-died-of-covid-19/

8. https://www.theguardian.com/world/2020/apr/18/nhs-frontline
-staff-may-refuse-to-work-over-lack-of-coronavirus-ppe-says-union
-unison

9. https://www.hulldailymail.co.uk/news/health/nursing
-nhs-staff-heroes-unhelpful-4088724

10. https://www.theguardian.com/world/2020/mar/06/gps-told
-to-switch-to-remote-consultations-to-combat-covid-19

11. https://www.dailymail.co.uk/news/article-9558165/Mail-Sunday
-leads-campaign-make-GPs-patients-face-face-again.html

12. https://www.spectator.co.uk/article/its-time-for-nhs-gps-to-stop
-hiding-behind-their-telephones/

13. https://www.dailymail.co.uk/news/article-10090001/The
-new-face-face-revolution-Sajid-Javid-launches-overhaul-GP-access
.html

14. https://www.theguardian.com/uk-news/2021/oct/10/nhs
-staff-face-rising-tide-of-abuse-from-patients-provoked-by-long
-waits

15. https://www.yorkshirepost.co.uk/news/politics/gps-hit-back-at
-out-of-touch-sajid-javid-after-health-secretary-demands-face-to-face
-appointments-return-3383071
16. https://www.manchestereveningnews.co.uk/news/greater-manchester
-news/what-happening-health-bosses-fury-21611733
17. https://www.legislation.gov.uk/ukpga/2022/31/contents/enacted
18. https://www.theguardian.com/society/2022/sep/01/nhs-vacancies
-in-england-at-staggering-new-high-as-almost-10-of-posts-empty
19. https://www.bma.org.uk/our-campaigns/consultant-campaigns
/pay/pay-pensions-and-ddrb-reform-for-consultants-in-england
20. https://www.theguardian.com/society/2022/nov/09/real-terms
-fall-in-uk-nurses-pay-is-part-of-wider-trend
21. https://www.theguardian.com/society/2022/sep/30/nhs-nurses
-not-eating-at-work-in-order-to-feed-their-children-survey-finds
22. https://www.bmj.com/content/373/bmj.n1461
23. https://www.theguardian.com/society/2022/feb/26/stressed
-nhs-staff-quit-at-record-rate-of-400-a-week-fuelling-fears-over
-care-quality
24. https://fullfact.org/health/what-is-naylor-review/
25. https://www.independent.co.uk/news/uk/politics/nhs-hospital
-land-secret-sale-tories-privatisation-sell-off-theresa-may-labour
-warning-medical-sites-a7885071.html
26. https://digital.nhs.uk/data-and-information/publications/statistical
/nhs-surplus-land/quarter-4-2021-22
27. https://www.ft.com/content/6f9f6f1f-e2d1-4646-b5ec
-7d704e45149e
28. https://www.theguardian.com/society/2021/aug/22/nhs-data-grab
-on-hold-as-millions-opt-out
29. Ibid.
30. https://www.instituteforgovernment.org.uk/blog/boris-johnson
-must-deliver-promised-plan-fix-social-care
31. https://www.theguardian.com/society/2022/sep/11/millions-uk
-patients-forced-private-nhs-waiting-lists

REFERENCES

32. https://www.theguardian.com/society/2022/mar/02/private-healthcare-boom-two-tier-system-uk

33. https://www.bma.org.uk/media/4316/bma-medical-staffing-report-in-england-july-2021.pdf

34. Ibid.

35. https://www.bbc.com/news/health-64189116

36. https://www.theguardian.com/commentisfree/2022/dec/08/people-in-pain-private-hospitals-nhs

37. https://www.independent.co.uk/news/uk/politics/coronavirus-uk-nhs-privatisation-hospital-survey-a9598826.html

38. https://www.itv.com/news/granada/2023-01-26/woman-87-who-could-not-afford-heating-died-from-hypothermia

39. https://www.telegraph.co.uk/politics/2023/01/14/public-support-nhs-strikes-soars-amid-warnings-put-lives-risk/

CHAPTER 5

1. https://www.ft.com/content/b0661cfe-3cf7-447f-862e-312f78aba36a; https://www.theguardian.com/society/2022/jun/29/nhs-privatisation-drive-linked-to-rise-in-avoidable-deaths-study-suggests

2. https://www.thelancet.com/journals/lanpub/article/PIIS2468-2667(22)00133-5/fulltext

3. https://www.opendemocracy.net/en/nhs-privatisation-health-social-care-treatable-deaths/; https://www.ox.ac.uk/news/2022-06-30-health-outsourcing-linked-higher-mortality-rate-oxford-study; https://www.bmj.com/content/377/bmj.o1612; https://www.bloomberg.com/news/articles/2022-06-29/privatizing-nhs-services-may-lead-to-declining-care-study-says

4. https://www.spectator.co.uk/article/are-we-falling-out-of-love-with-the-nhs/

5. https://www.bbc.com/news/health-62986347

6. https://iea.org.uk/about-us

7. https://www.bbc.com/news/health-62986347

8. http://www.docsnotcops.co.uk/about/

9. https://www.practitionerhealth.nhs.uk

10. https://doctors-in-distress.org.uk

11. https://www.bbc.com/news/uk-england-london-62348826

12. https://www.theguardian.com/society/2022/jun/14/rundown-nhs-hospitals-have-become-a-danger-to-patients-warn-health-chiefs

13. https://www.nhsconfed.org/news/lack-capital-funding-risking-patient-safety-and-impeding-waiting-list-recovery-new-poll-nhs

14. https://www.theguardian.com/politics/2022/oct/25/nhs-hospital-trusts-paying-hundreds-of-millions-in-interest-to-private-firms

15. Ibid.

16. https://www.newstatesman.com/spotlight/healthcare/2022/05/pfi-repayments-are-costing-some-hospitals-twice-as-much-as-drugs

17. https://www.theguardian.com/society/2013/sep/18/nhs-records-system-10bn

18. https://www.wired.co.uk/article/babylon-disrupted-uk-health-system-then-left

19. https://www.nationalarchives.gov.uk/education/resources/attlees-britain/beveridge-report/